Spirituality and Personhood in Dementia

Spirituality and Personhood in Dementia

Edited by
Albert Jewell

Jessica Kingsley *Publishers*
London and Philadelphia

Material in the second half of Chapter 1 from Hawley and Jewell
2009 is reproduced by permission of MHA Care Group.
Material in Chapter 4 is reproduced by permission of Shinko Igaku Publishing.
Excerpts on p.59 and p.63 from TMK Productions and Memory Bridge 2007 are
reproduced by permission of Michael Verde, Memory Bridge Foundation.
Extract on pp.53–54 from Ignatieff 1992 is reproduced by
permission of © Guardian News & Media Ltd 2010.
Material in Chapter 8 from Green 2007 is reproduced by
permission of the British Psychological Society.
Verse from Carter 1963 on p.107 is reproduced by permission of Stainer & Bell Ltd, London, England.
Figure 13.1 and extract on p.144 from Lloyd 2004 are reproduced by permission of Geriaction.
Figure 13.2 on p.146 from Lloyd 2004 is reproduced by permission of Hawker Publications.
Verse on p.150 is from 'As Long As I Have Music'. Words by Nancy Price and Don Besig.
Music by Don Besig. Copyright © 1986 by Shawnee Press, Inc. International Copyright
Secured. All Rights Reserved. Reproduced by permission of Hal Leonard Corporation.
Extract on p.157 from Arthey 1997 is reproduced by permission of Vin Arthey.
Verses in Chapter 15 from the New English Bible, © Oxford University Press and Cambridge
University Press 1961, 1970, are reproduced by permission of Cambridge University Press.

First published in 2011
by Jessica Kingsley Publishers
116 Pentonville Road
London N1 9JB, UK
and
400 Market Street, Suite 400
Philadelphia, PA 19106, USA

www.jkp.com

Copyright © Jessica Kingsley Publishers 2011

Library of Congress Cataloging in Publication Data
A CIP catalog record for this book is available from the Library of Congress

British Library Cataloguing in Publication Data
A CIP catalogue record for this book is available from the British Library

ISBN 978 1 84905 154 5

Printed and bound in Great Britain

CONTENTS

PREFACE

Albert Jewell

This is the third book relating to spirituality in old age that I have edited since 1999, all published by Jessica Kingsley Publishers. The first was *Spirituality and Ageing* (Jewell 1999). The second was *Ageing, Spirituality and Well-being* (Jewell 2004), which brought together major contributions made at Durham International Conference on Ageing, Spirituality and Well-being in 2002. In the first volume, 5 out of the 17 chapters dealt directly with dementia; in the second it was 2 out of 14. Such a distribution was deliberate in light of the fact that only some 30 per cent of people are likely to develop the dementias that most characterise old age. It seemed important to maintain a sense of proportion. This book, the third of the trilogy, however, is devoted exclusively to dementia and its implications for spirituality and personhood.

My personal route into the subject has three connected sources. It will be noticed that the chapters throughout the book resound with references to the late Professor Tom Kitwood, whom I met 15 years ago at a training course held at Woodbrooke, the Quaker study centre in Birmingham. He made a huge impression and conversations lasted late into the night. I remember especially how he asked us to divide into pairs, one partner simulating an older person with dementia and the other their companion or carer. Much insight was gained from this role-play session. Later, he movingly described William Penn, who in his latter years in America was in advanced dementia and yet was still venerated by his community and given due dignity as their leader. Tom spoke to me of how he had long before become disillusioned as an evangelical mission partner in Africa and had grown out of a dogmatic faith into a much broader spirituality. My own spiritual journey was not dissimilar. Kitwood is credited with revolutionising the way people with dementia are perceived, though it has to be admitted that actual practice for the most part still lags far behind theory. There is a sense in which this book can be regarded as a *Festschrift* in his honour, and Clive Baldwin and John Swinton in their chapters provide valuable 'Kitwood critiques'.

The second source lies in the work of MHA Care Group (formerly Methodist Homes for the Aged) whose pastoral director I became in 1994. MHA warmly embraced Kitwood's view of the importance of 'the person, not the problem' (Kitwood 1997a). Person-centred care and the need to sustain each individual's spirituality became enshrined in the homes and schemes run by MHA. It was my privilege to work with others to produce a spirituality model which was capable of embracing all in MHA's care, including those with the perceived diminishments of dementia. This approach was encapsulated in MHA's staff training DVD, 'Nourishing the Inner Being' (MHA 2002), and has been described in my introduction to the book *Ageing, Spirituality and Well-being* (Jewell 2004).

The third source lies in my post-retirement life during which I became the secretary of the Christian Council on Ageing Dementia Group and editor of its Dementia Newsletter. This brought me into contact with an expanding circle of people researching and working in the dementia field, who have served to challenge stereotypes, change attitudes and demonstrate what is achievable in the care of those with dementia. Several have contributed chapters to the present volume. To them I am very grateful, but most of all to Tom Kitwood who brought hope and light into a dark corner of human experience.

There is a further commonality in the three books I have edited. It is all too easy to presume a dominant Christian culture but today in most Western countries many religions and cultures intermingle and secularism is dominant. Whilst it was not possible to include chapters covering every faith community in the books I have edited, in the first volume there were contributions from the Jewish faith and on British Hindus, Sikhs and Muslims; Eastern perspectives also featured in the second book, in a chapter written by Dr Krishna Mohan. In the present volume, several of the writers, notably Padmaprabha Dalby, John Killick, Paul Green and Brian Allen, urge the relevance of Buddhist insights (especially that of 'mindfulness') in understanding people with dementia, not least their capacity to live in the present moment, and Susan McFadden refers to the Taoist idea of *wu wei* ('life in tune with the universe'). Malcolm Goldsmith deals specifically with the non-religious living in a secular society, and all the writers are fully aware that 'spirituality' is far wider and more inclusive than 'religion'. Throughout, the emphasis of this book is on spirituality rather than theology and on experience rather than dogma.

The contributions fall into several sections and the book has been put together in what some may see as 'reverse order'. The more theoretical, conceptual and philosophical chapters have been placed at the end. The early chapters have been written from an intensely personal point of view. These are then followed by authors writing about their research, and by practitioners, including trainers. It is hoped that the book will be of particular value to those responsible for the care of older people, and to the general reader who has a concern for people living with dementia.

CHAPTER 1

Introduction

Albert Jewell

A PERSONAL JOURNEY

For the first half of my pastoral ministry I have to say that I lived largely in ignorance of dementia. This was in part due to the fact that my concentration was upon children and young people. It is also true that older people with dementia tended either to be found tucked away in the back room of the family home, where they were often regarded as harmlessly eccentric, or living long-term in the large out-of-town psychiatric hospitals that were a feature of the post-war period in Britain.

My education developed apace from the mid-1980s. I well remember, after several months in a new church, discovering that the mother of a very active church family lived in such a hospital. Although she had herself previously been a live-wire in church and community, now she was not mentioned at all. When I visited her, I was horrified at what I found in her locked ward. Patients were lying moaning on the floor in foetal positions or confined within armchairs from which they could not move. Faeces and rubbish littered the floor and the noise was harrowing. I am sure that staff members were doing their best, but theirs was a work of restraint and containment, and the lack of humanity or any sense of purpose was palpable. I felt that there was little I could do in the pandemonium and was glad to get out of the ward after just a few minutes trying to communicate with the elderly woman I had come to visit – who in any case did not know me.

Later I moved to a church in another part of the country, full of very active older people, ministering effectively to the needs of that age group through a day centre and a support group for those with dementia and their families. I also served as chaplain at a hospital with two psycho-geriatric wards. I have a vivid memory of conducting a Sunday afternoon service during which one patient approached me in mid-sermon and gradually wound her very long scarf round me from the feet up until I resembled an

Egyptian mummy. I should have realised that she was signalling she had had enough of my talking!

In one of the geriatric wards I used to move round and sit next to every patient in order to engage them in conversation or just spend a brief time of quiet with them. There was one man I tended to avoid because he seemed always to be waving his arms around in a highly threatening manner. One day the staff nurse on duty invited me into her office and asked me why it was that I greeted each patient personally but just gave a peremptory wave towards this one man. I explained my fear of getting too close in case I got hit, whereupon she asked whether I had ever thought that he acted as he did when he saw me enter the ward because he knew that he would be to all intents and purposes ignored. Moreover, she explained, it might interest me to know that he was a renowned Oxford University professor who happened to suffer from Huntington's disease. Thereafter I changed my practice, but sadly the man died quite soon afterwards.

Visiting her husband, who spent regular periods of respite care at that hospital, was a woman who had experienced a hard life coping with him and his periodic violence. She found a real refuge in writing poetry. She used to bring her husband to the evening service at our church because it was less 'busy' than the morning one and the congregation much smaller. I used to welcome the couple so enthusiastically that I tended to over-excite the husband and needed to learn that what they were both seeking most of all was a peaceful space, a time of refreshment and renewal.

As pastoral director of MHA Care Group I of course encountered growing numbers of older people at various stages of dementia. I can truly say that my most exhilarating experiences took place within the dementia unit of one of MHA's residential homes. The individuals living there had led fascinating and varied lives. It was always such a hive of activity and overt happiness that it lifted up the heart of any visitor. It had a small, dedicated staff team with whom the residents could form quite close relationships. In fact, those in the adjoining 'ordinary' care home became rather jealous of the evident *joie de vivre* of their near neighbours!

Following my retirement from full-time ministry my dementia 'education' continued. I had the rather unusual experience of visiting a former ministerial colleague who at that time was resident in a care home for people with dementia. It was sad to find a man of such brilliant mind who had become so confused. The home found him difficult to cope with because he wandered restlessly and was prone to get into the wrong bed. He did his best to communicate when I called, but asked me the same questions over and over again and could not retain my replies. He was at an advanced stage in his dementia and died soon afterwards. However, I shall never forget him saying with great sadness, 'I'm losing my marbles, and I know it. I find it very depressing.' It is hardly surprising that the two conditions, dementia and depression, tend to go together. This is what lends significance to the chapters by Paul Green and Murray Lloyd in this book (Chapters 8 and 13 respectively).

Such has been my personal journey of discovery and growth of understanding in relation to dementia.

SPIRITUALITY

This book is concerned with the degree to which spirituality may be sustained and personhood preserved in the face of dementia – indeed, with the inter-relatedness of all three.

In the first book I edited (Jewell 1999, p.14) I argued that spirituality 'can be interpreted so broadly as to lose any distinctiveness or so narrowly as to appear to exclude large numbers of people'. Spirituality should certainly not be restricted to a narrowly Christian version. I would want to maintain that every person is a spiritual person, whether or not they recognise it. However, some more precise definition is helpful. I would see 'the spiritual' as including those intangibles in life which are nevertheless of great significance to us. Such would incorporate principles and beliefs, values, the aesthetic and a sense of awe. In particular, finding meaning and purpose in life would seem to be very important; meaning being primarily retrospective, purpose prospective (Jewell 2010). For some their spirituality will include belief in a god or divine force, for others not. Julian Hughes in his chapter (Chapter 18) sees spirituality in terms of the transcendent – that which goes beyond the physical/material – and regards it as 'a non-negotiable ingredient of personhood'.

I have subsequently come to realise that relationships are an all-important aspect of spirituality – a recurrent theme in this book. A general consensus does seem to emerge amongst its authors. In Chapter 10 Gaynor Hammond majors on the relationship aspect, defined in terms of family, friends, community, the natural world and God. Susan McFadden (Chapter 9) takes a similar view, seeing spirituality as 'seeking sacred meaning in relationships with God, other people, the natural and human-created environment, and within the self'. Elizabeth MacKinlay (Chapter 4) defines spirituality in terms of finding meaning and hope, and also in the capacity to respond to the numinous. From this brief excursus it is possible to discern three main components of spirituality: a sense of relatedness, a sense of purpose or meaning in life and a sense of transcendence. To over-simplify, dementia tends to affect relationships and challenge any cognitive sense of meaning, but does not deprive people of responding to what moves them deeply, often in a more spontaneous way than those without the condition.

PERSONHOOD

It is all too easy to make the misguided assumption that people with dementia have ceased to be 'persons' in the full sense of that word. So long as that assumption is made, it is hardly surprising if it becomes a self-fulfilling prophecy: through the assumptions and attitudes of others they can so easily be further marginalised, rather than positively included within mainstream human society, and defining personhood in terms of individual identity risks seeing them in isolation from others. Clive Baldwin's chapter (Chapter 17) is especially helpful in this respect, and in Chapter 6 Padmaprabha Dalby helpfully recalls Kitwood's definition of personhood as 'a standing or status that is bestowed on one human being, by others, in the context of relationship and social being' (Kitwood 1997a, p.8). Baldwin also proposes a fluid rather than fixed view of personhood: an ongoing process of becoming rather than something fixed or static.

I would argue that there are some seven essential aspects to our identity/ personhood which may be affected in dementia but which can be conserved if due care is exercised by other people.

Memory

Memory is what gives us our continuity through time as persons and we recognise that we are in large measure the product of our past experience. In most forms of dementia it is the short-term memory that is affected first and worst, whilst more distant memories can survive relatively unimpaired for a long time. Strangely, at least in the earlier stages of dementia, longer-term memory can appear to be intensified, so that the person with dementia may well not remember what they have just eaten for lunch, whilst being able to recall in great detail events and people from the distant past. It is almost as if much of the intervening trivial clutter has been cleared away, leaving in sharper relief some of the more significant things from a person's past – from which, indeed, they derive their personhood.

The Leeds-based Faith in Elderly People project encourages older people to make use of 'memory boxes' (Treetops 1999), adapting a practice pioneered by Barnardo's in the care of children from families where one or both parents were suffering from HIV/AIDS and likely to leave them as orphans. A memory box is a gathered collection of very personal things that have been important to a person over the years and which help to identify who they are. It could comprise photographs (provided that they are properly labelled), books, music, prized presents, certificates and awards, favoured scents, objects of religious significance, etc. Tactile objects can be particularly evocative. Indeed, many an older person's living room and bedroom contain an abundance of such things, which can provide a focus for meaningful conversation for visitors and carers. I suggest that it is never too early to begin putting a memory box together!

Several of the contributors to this book stress the present moment as the most significant time dimension for persons with dementia.

Reason

Human beings are *homo sapiens*. We have the capacity to reason and work things out. The damage caused by dementia means that a person's cerebral functions are progressively impaired. It is as if something gets in the way between thinking the thought and carrying it out or communicating it to someone else. Stroke sufferers can face similar problems. It adds greatly to the frustration of the person with dementia if other people lack patience and appear to treat them as if they are no longer a thinking human being! John Swinton in Chapter 16 argues cogently that 'dementia is as much a relational disability as it is a physical or neurological one'.

Feelings

We are emotional as well as rational beings and these two aspects of our personhood need to be kept in balance. People with dementia continue to experience the full gamut of human feelings. Indeed, their expression is often intensified through a process of 'disinhibition', lowering rational restraints sometimes to the point of causing embarrassment to others. However, honestly expressed and sensitively interpreted, they are an enormous aid to effective communication. Body language can express what verbal communication often conceals.

Gaynor Hammond in Chapter 10 presents a training module which gives due priority to understanding and engaging with the emotions of people with dementia, and several of the contributors value music in particular as facilitating their expression.

Senses

Human beings are sensual creatures. The trouble is that we tend to rely too much on mouth-to-ear communication. However, many older people suffer from hearing deficiencies, and these multiply the difficulties for people with dementia. Sight is equally important, and again, many older people, including those with dementia, are visually impaired to some degree. This means that the evocative senses of smell and taste can assume a greater significance, and touch (appropriately used) is the most important of all in dispelling isolation, as John Killick illustrates in Chapter 5.

Choice

The Swiss doctor and theologian Paul Tournier (1957) maintained that to live is to choose. This is embedded in the Judeo-Christian doctrine of humanity from the first chapters of Genesis onwards. The corollary is that to reduce choice diminishes personhood.

In a recent book on decision-making arising from an international multidisciplinary workshop (O'Connor and Purves 2009) the issues of capability, capacity and competence have been well addressed, largely in connection with legal and ethical decisions but also with reference to the use of support services. The thrust of the present book is more general (though Wendy Shiels in Chapter 11 does deal with advance directives), but no less important. As with others whose abilities are impaired, people with dementia are so often caught up in the 'does he take sugar?' syndrome, where quite 'ordinary' everyday choices or decisions are offered to carers, or otherwise made without reference to the actual person concerned. However, people with dementia are still able to make choices and thereby preserve their dignity, provided they are given time and not addressed in too complex a way. Marianne Talbot describes in Chapter 3 how she strove to preserve her mother's ability to choose.

Skills

Creativity lies at the heart of being human. Again, in the Judeo-Christian tradition this can be traced to the concept that humanity has been made in the image of a creator God. It is too easily assumed that skills inevitably disappear for people with dementia – and indeed, it is distressing, in the later stages, if they 'forget' how to carry out even such basic tasks as feeding and washing themselves. However, there is evidence that many skills, especially artistic and musical abilities, are retained at great length and even that, in a suitably stimulating and encouraging environment, new skills can be acquired despite the manifest diminishments of dementia. A striking example is that of the American artist William de Kooning, who painted some of his greatest pictures in his eighties and nineties, after developing Alzheimer's disease. Several of the chapters in this book, notably those by Harriet Mowat (Chapter 7), Susan McFadden (Chapter 9), Gaynor Hammond (Chapter 10) and Murray Lloyd (Chapter 13), illustrate the importance of these creative skills, Mowat making a suggestive link with *homo ludens*.

Relationships

The central doctrine of Christianity is the Trinity, the understanding that God is in essence relational. It is maintained that the same is true of human beings made in God's image. They have not been created to remain isolated individuals. As already argued, in large measure we derive and preserve our personhood from relationships with other people. For people with dementia, continued bonding with family members and old friends is very important, and they are also well capable of forming new significant relationships with other dementia sufferers, professional carers and regular visitors. Family members may find this difficult to accept, especially when they themselves appear no longer to be recognised. Friends, neighbours and former colleagues may feel that they do not know what to say and cease to visit. Regrettably, churches and other faith groups can also effectively cut themselves off from people with dementia and their families because of lack of understanding and empathy. This, however, only compounds their sense of isolation and, for those to whom their faith has been of great importance, sense of abandonment by God.

Elizabeth MacKinlay's chapter (Chapter 4) is a moving testimony to her continuing personal and spiritual relationship with Christine Bryden, and Padmaprabha Dalby shows in Chapter 6 how such relationships are reciprocal in the case of individuals whose spirituality is based upon love, generosity and altruism.

IMPLICATIONS

These threatened aspects of personhood have important implications with regard to communicating with people with dementia, care-giving, worship, and the theological assumptions or models generally favoured in Christian communities.

Communication

From childhood, human beings thrive through communication and are diminished without it or when it is restricted. Alistair McFadyen, in his densely argued book *Call to Personhood* (1990), takes the view (as does Brian Allen in Chapter 14 of this volume) that we are essentially 'dialogical' rather than 'analogical' as human beings. Our personhood is 'sedimented' from our earliest years through communication with our significant others, and it will continue to be nourished or diminished by the quality of communication in our adult and later years.

One of the most significant recent developments in dementia care has been the development of the person-centred approach, pioneered by Tom Kitwood (1997a), into a more explicitly relationship-centred model which recognises the importance of family, friends and community (including faith communities) alongside the contribution of professional carers (Woods, Keady and Seddon 2008; Whitman 2010).

The poet John Killick has recorded his conversations with individuals at various stages of dementia and is convinced that most reveal a desperate desire to communicate verbally, alongside a sense of disempowerment because so few people seem to have the time and patience to facilitate it. He writes: 'Occasionally when I have been sitting with these silent ones I have been privileged to witness "the clouds part" and I have been vouchsafed words which interpret the muteness, and do so with incredible insight' (Killick 1997, p.15).

People with dementia have considerable difficulty in recalling and articulating the right words at the right time. However, as already argued, communication is not entirely dependent upon actual language: body language plays a large part and communication can continue through signs such as nods, taps and squeezes for 'yes' and 'no'. Much practical advice is given by Malcolm Goldsmith in his carefully researched book, *Hearing the Voices of People with Dementia* (1996), and in the leaflet *Visiting People with Dementia* (2008) produced by MHA and the Christian Council on Ageing (MHA/CCOA). Both Killick and Goldsmith contribute powerful chapters in this book (Chapters 5 and 15 respectively).

Appropriate care

Throughout the government's National Dementia Strategy consultation process held in England by the Department of Health during 2008, which concentrated in the main upon early diagnosis and access to services, it was continually pointed out by respondents that any improvement in the delivery of care services would depend in large measure upon the presence of well-trained staff. Lip service is now paid to person-centred care, but actual practice can lag far behind. Here, the chapters by Gaynor Hammond (Chapter 10), Wendy Shiels (Chapter 11), Margaret Goodall (Chapter 12) and Brian Allen (Chapter 14) have much to contribute.

Worship

Human beings of all religions often feel that they 'find themselves' and sustain their personhood through a relationship with God nurtured by prayer and worship. The experience of dementia, as recorded for example by Robert Davis (1992), can appear to open up a dark abyss in which God seems to be absent and personal prayer almost impossible. It is not easy to 'sing the Lord's song' in such a strange land, the land of forgetfulness. Prayer with visitors and corporate worship, therefore, can be vital. Indeed, in worship by people with dementia there can be an immediacy, joyfulness and trust which one could wish present in every congregation!

However, leading worship in such a context is quite demanding. Practical help is available in the leaflet *Worship with People with Dementia*, jointly produced by MHA and CCOA (2006). In Chapter 9 of this volume Susan McFadden shows how worship with people with dementia can be playful, creative and truly inclusive; Gaynor Hammond writes in Chapter 10 about worship in care homes; and Harriet Mowat in Chapter 7 extols the value of what she terms 'expressive space'.

Theology

It is a sobering thought that the model or framework of theology that Christians (whether consciously or not) adopt, and which undergirds their attitudes and practices, can have the unfortunate effect of further marginalising people with dementia. The same may be true in the case of other religions.

Malcolm Goldsmith (1999) has drawn attention to some popular models that are distinctly unhelpful. These include a model dependent upon the living memory of the relationship of God with his people. In the case of people with dementia it is necessary for the faith community to remember with and for them. Similarly, the Roman Catholic and Wesleyan models of sanctification, which emphasise growth towards that 'perfect love' which is God's essence, are of little value to those whose personhood and life experience are being fragmented and set back by dementia. Many models stress the making, developing and deepening of relationships variously with God the Father, Jesus and the Holy Spirit, and with one's fellow-believers and fellow-human beings. Once more, this is not helpful to those who feel their relationships with other people threatened and whose sense of God's presence may have been progressively eroded. The challenge remains for churches to work at continuing relationships with people with dementia.

To these theological models one might add 'the Protestant work ethic' model. It is rather odd that this should have developed and become so entrenched within many Christian faith communities which historically have stressed that salvation is by God's grace alone, to which we need simply to open ourselves through faith. However, in practice nowadays most Protestant denominations are activist and seem to place great store on working out, even 'earning', our salvation by what we do and achieve. As a consequence people tend to be valued for what they contribute in the service of the church rather than for their own sake. People with advanced dementia can 'do' little, perhaps nothing at all. Will they still be cherished within a Protestant work ethic culture?

In urging the Church to discover a more appropriate and inclusive model, Goldsmith (1999) proposes an alternative, which he terms 'remembered and valued by God'. This model has its roots in God's unconditional love for the human beings he has created, the extent of which is seen in the death and resurrection of Christ. The lines of the hymn, 'Nothing in my hand I bring, Simply to thy cross I cling', apply to all alike. Such a model shifts attention away from ourselves (what we believe, remember or do) and onto God's mercy and love. It reminds us that even when we forget him, God still remembers us and always will. This is the model, Goldsmith urges, that ultimately brings good news to the person with dementia – as to everyone.

GROUNDS FOR HOPE

There are some further shafts of light in what can seem a very dark landscape. Eileen Shamy (2003, p.20) records how, after her mother had ceased to communicate meaningfully for some time in the care home where she spent her last days, she sat up, looked her daughter in the eye and declared, 'God never forgets us. Remember that, dear!' Such moments of illumination are not uncommon in the later stages of dementia, as Julian Hughes notes in Chapter 18. It is as if a shaft of light has suddenly illuminated the individual and for a short while reveals their essential personhood.

In Chapter 3 Marianne Talbot gives testimony to the perseverance of her mother's personhood even as her dementia increased.

The study by Dr David Snowden of 678 Notre Dame Roman Catholic sisters in the USA (2001) has also proved most revealing. With the permission of the order, he carried out autopsies which showed that some sisters whose brains displayed all the features of advanced dementia had shown little or no trace of it in their lives in their community. He considered the various factors that might account for this sustaining of normality (genes, diet, lifelong employment, etc.) and concluded that the explanation could lie only in more intangible 'spiritual' factors, such as their regular liturgical pattern of life and the strength of their corporate life and fellowship. This, in the view expressed by Clive Baldwin in Chapter 17, is their 'defining community'. There are obvious lessons here, for those who have ears to hear, within the corporate life of local churches. As Shamy writes: 'Personhood cannot be taken from us because it is God-given' (2003, p.129).

A refreshing development in publishing has been the number of books written by individuals with dementia or in conjunction with their family carers (Bryden 2005; Bryden and MacKinlay 2008; Davis 1992). Those who can speak most eloquently about their continuing, indeed developing, personhood are those who experience dementia first-hand. This is where Chapter 2 by Dr Daphne Wallace is so valuable, she being both an old age psychiatrist and someone with recently diagnosed vascular dementia who continues to find sustaining purpose in life.

In her informative but rather bleak account of caring for her mother-in-law in advanced dementia, Andrea Gillies (2009, p.351) concludes that 'It's time to stop reading the dementia books'. It is hoped that this book majoring on spirituality and personhood will prove an exception and engender a real measure of hope, albeit always tinged with due realism.

CHAPTER 2

Maintaining a Sense of Personhood in Dementia

A Personal View

Daphne Wallace

The image of a UK care home in most people's minds is often the complete antithesis of 'person-centred': old people sitting round a room, dozing the day away. This ageist stereotype offers a very depressing picture of what it is going to be like for them, and so denial comes to the fore. Until recently people with dementia were diagnosed relatively late and were often looked after in a very impersonal way. In the past almost everyone known to have this illness was in the late stages of dementia and almost always to be seen in institutions, sitting round the room in chairs, sleeping a lot, not interacting with people round about them, unresponsive and disengaged. Such classic images led to the residents being thought of as non-persons. This is not, of course, how the late stages of Alzheimer's disease should be experienced, but that is how it has appeared and it is certainly the image that many people retain.

Some people want to deny the personhood of someone with a severe learning disability. Old age and disability may be felt to impair the person. Similarly, severe dementia is seen by many as destroying the person. Denial of the person precludes a relationship. I have worked over the years with many people with both conditions. I have always seen them as persons and have come to have a great respect for many struggling with such difficulties. I have tried throughout my working life and since my retirement to promote such ideas. I have also been involved with several people who have contributed extensively to the understanding of these principles.

Paul Tournier (1898–1986) wrote about the person in medicine (1957). A Swiss physician and writer, Tournier was an advocate of the integrative approach to medicine, psychology and pastoral counselling. He wrote many books about the doctor's relationship with patients and their personal and spiritual problems: medicine of the whole person. He was the founder of an international organisation, *Médecine de la Personne*, of which I am a member in its British and International groups. Tournier emphasised that developing spiritual sensitivity in a therapeutic relationship was essential. This relied on Martin Buber's concept of the 'I–Thou' relationship rather than the impersonal 'I–It' encounter (Buber 1958). What Tournier commended and practised was 'an integrative, person-centred medicine that considers psychospiritual as well as biosocial aspects of patient care, and in particular recognizes the healing potential of a caring relationship' (Cox, Campbell and Fulford 2007, p.44).

Tom Kitwood, whom I knew well, wrote about 'personhood' and people with dementia. His seminal work, carried on by the Bradford Dementia Group since his death, showed how the behaviour of those with dementia was not due to the illness so much as to the way society regarded them. In his scientific papers (Kitwood 1993; Kitwood and Bredin 1992a) Kitwood sets out his theories in relation to dementia care, emphasising that personhood should be seen in social rather than individual terms. My understanding has always been that, without seeing the person as a whole, we fail to appreciate the interaction between the underlying personality, physical health, life history, social psychology and the neurological damage to the brain.

Another important influence on my thinking is Julian Hughes, who considers different accounts of what it means to be a person and concludes:

> However, if we can argue that being minded and having memories is not just to do with what is going on in the head, then we can argue that neither is being a person. Hence we are still persons if we have severe dementia. At least, we can still retain our personhood if the external circumstances (psychosocial environment or the ways in which we are treated) are right. Hence the importance of 'person-centred care', since this always implies a broad view of what it is to be a person. (Hughes 2008, p.126)

I have also been involved since its foundation in the Dementia Group (formerly Dementia Working Group) of the Christian Council on Ageing, an inter-denominational group concerned with the spiritual needs of people with dementia. Despite the fact that spiritual care is now recognised as part of good integrated care in any National Health Service and other care settings, it is often ignored or inadequately provided. This is thought of by many as having to do with religion. If the person concerned has a religious faith, then indeed their spiritual needs include maintenance of their faith practice. People with no religious faith, however, also have spiritual needs. Spiritual wellbeing is relevant and important. Attention to spiritual needs leads to a better quality of life. Meeting them is not an add-on 'icing on the cake' but an integral part of whole person care. Spiritual care involves giving time and concentrated attention to an individual, listening carefully to what they say, ensuring their wellbeing and attending to their religious needs if they have a faith.

My own sense of personhood has always included my relationship with God. Over the years I have varied in how spontaneously I am able to express my beliefs. As a student I was involved in the 'Tell Scotland Movement', which ran missions in Scotland, including Glenrothes and Leith, in which I participated. I learnt to stand in a pulpit and speak, with a real sense of being led by the Spirit. We also knocked on doors, which required some confidence-building. Since then I have varied in confidence in outward profession of faith, but my faith has not dimmed and has always been in the background in my work and family life. I do not feel that I have special enlightenment as a Christian psychiatrist but believe that I am a better psychiatrist than I would be without my Christian faith.

So that is where I found myself and my ideas in 2005. I am now well into the 'older adult age range', having retired from the health service over ten years ago. Five years after my retirement I did a part-time locum to help former colleagues. After finishing my five-month stint I realised that I was not coping too well and noticed some particular deficiencies in function that I had been accustomed to recognising in my patients. After discussion with some close colleagues I saw my GP and a referral went to the local neurologist. He arranged a scan and an assessment by a neuro-psychologist. These eventually confirmed that I had changes in my scan and functioning that were indicative of very early small-vessel vascular dementia. This fitted with a strong family history of vascular disease. I was put on appropriate medication for the vascular disease and it was agreed that I would be followed up by my GP when the neurologist moved to Australia.

Reactions to the diagnosis were very varied, especially amongst friends and colleagues. Some were dismissive, saying things like 'We all have that, it's your age', or 'I've never been able to do that', or worse, 'You're doing too much, you need to slow down'. However, I know that, like my mother, I have always packed a lot into a day and still do. If I slowed down as suggested I feel I would grind to a halt with depression. I cannot change the basic person I am. Such reactions felt very diminishing of me both as a person and professionally. Other friends were empathic, realising that there was an element of grief and bereavement as I reassessed my future plans and prospects, in particular the effect of finding in myself the changes I had seen in others in my work.

I have had to adjust to a sense of loss and acceptance. There has been a subtle change in my attitude to the future and practical adjustments day to day. Once I came to a sense of acceptance I realised that I needed to have some expert follow-up but my GP at first did not feel that this was needed. Eventually we agreed that the GP would write to a local consultant for older people, and I now have six-monthly checks, as well as my cardio-vascular checks from the GP clinic. This has enabled me to be referred for neuro-psychological reassessment which has shown, after three-and-a-half years, that there has been only minimal change in my functioning, thus ruling out, as far as is possible, any additional pathology.

I enjoy working with friends I have made in the 'Living with Dementia' group I now belong to. We all accept each other as we are and have a sense of camaraderie which is empowering. We are fortunate. So many people with early dementia find themselves in a very different world. Consequently, they are perplexed and frustrated at the reaction of others – whether denial or acceptance, but then diminishment as they are assumed to be unable to do things which they can still do, even if more slowly. They may get a diagnosis, which is often a relief, but then no follow-up until they have problems and need 'services'.

Since this change in my life several basic questions seem to me to arise. Who am I? What is at the heart of who I am? What is it that needs to be preserved? Is my personhood fixed or is it continuously evolving? Does the person change with age? There are many ways of describing a person: it may be in terms of what the person does, believes, is, or what is important to them. I believe that all these aspects are significant, but the balance may change over a lifetime. An old friend of mine used to emphasise the change that he felt was needed – from 'doing' to 'being' (Wainwright 2001, published posthumously). He also wrote a poem in which he talked about his sense of diminishment but also the sustaining power of his faith.

What are the aspects of my personality that are important to the preservation of my personhood? Following a discussion in school when I was 11 years old, about which subjects to study at O-level, we were asked what we wanted to be when we left school. I answered 'a nurse'. My teacher replied with her own question, 'Have you ever thought of being a doctor?' The answer of course was 'no' but that became my single-minded goal. This required staying power when we moved to another area where the school had a limited science tradition. Some of my determination is that said to be characteristic of the small person! I certainly get my resourcefulness from my mother and I like to think that I have the warmth I knew in both parents, especially my father. When I qualified in medicine my colleagues described me as 'a professional athlete of the tongue'. Like my mother, I like to be active but I hope that over the years I have learnt to listen effectively as well as speak.

It is important to me that people understand what things matter to me. I am always busy but that is how I like it. I have many leisure interests. Eventually some may be ruled out, as angina has ruled out skiing. Music is especially important to me. I cannot at present imagine life without participation in music, though regrettably the instruments I used to play are now largely neglected. I enjoy cooking and dancing, although the opportunities for my first love, Scottish country dancing, are infrequent. I take after my mother in enjoying creative arts and crafts, especially sewing, painting and drawing. I like people and am interested in them. However, time is always short and I wish I had more hours in the day.

Some of my previous skills are diminished. I can no longer do arithmetic, which was never a problem in the past. My visual memory used to be exceptionally good – now it is just average. Words sometimes escape me, which makes writing hard and can interfere with conversations. I tend to trip over or bump into things, with bruises to show for it. I knock over glasses and other things on tables. All these are due not to impaired vision but to sluggish responses to visual clues.

I cannot deny that there are times when I feel overwhelmed and have moments of apprehension about the future. I am content with the past and what I have shared with others. The sharing goes on. I feel frustration at the things that become more difficult, including the vagaries of my computer. However, I am able to recognise what still goes on and my contribution to it.

I am still actively involved in parish life and the local village community where we live. My faith is not dimmed and I continue to write and speak in a small way on spiritual matters. Spontaneous prayer or 'words' are now more difficult; the skills honed on the streets of Leith are hampered by the searching for words that I am becoming used to. People ask me how my faith helps me. Others ask if what has happened to me brings anger or doubts. I felt the expected sadness and sense of loss when I first realised what was happening. More recently, however, I feel that what I am experiencing is something to work with, to turn into something that I can use to benefit others.

I have a real sense of God being with me on a journey. I try, like a good friend of ours with physical limitations, to feel it is a challenge that God is working on with me, rather than a 'punishment' or a 'trial' due to failures on my part.

In some ways I am still evolving as a person. I now give high priority to at least one aspect of music – I sing in more than one choir. I try to give priority to time spent with my husband and to developing our joint activities, together with contact with my family. I try to avoid more administrative activities, though sometimes they are hard to avoid! I use my experience and skills to try to increase understanding of the person with dementia and to spread knowledge of good attitudes and practice. I remain involved with the organisations I was associated with previously, related to person-centred care and dementia. In the years since the initiation of the National Dementia Strategy I have been very involved in various ways during its preparation and implementation.

My husband and I cannot know how much will be sustained in the coming years. We do not know in what way things will change. What I am certain of is that, however much these parts of my life may be impaired or curtailed, I will still be a person with a special past, with feelings, not just a shell 'sans everything'. I will not like tea. I will still love music, however imperfect my participation. Should life in my own home become unsustainable, I have long-held views about what the experience of care should be. Care should be person-centred and responsive to need. We have to remember that what others perceive as needed may be different from the needs felt by those cared for. Human beings are infinitely variable and therefore their needs are not easily predicted, so individual packages are the best way to meet those needs. I hope that this sort of care will be available to me, whether at home or in a care setting.

What will matter to me, if and when I become more dependent, will be my personal integrity and self-esteem, a sense of belonging and sufficient independence. I will want some influence over life, with control and choice and a sense of security, both financial and environmental.

My faith has provided a constant sustaining force. I retain a sense of journeying through whatever life presents with support from God travelling by my side. Throughout, my personhood is continually evolving with new directions based on experience and changing perspectives which can continue to maintain a sense of self. Although our problems differ I have made many new friends amongst those also living with dementia, who are all interesting and varied persons. We all know that late stages may be different and difficult but we intend to LIVE with our diagnosis, whatever the future holds.

CHAPTER 3

A Carer's Perspective

Marianne Talbot

'I wouldn't want to live with any of you!' Mum said whenever the subject of ageing came up. Dad wanted to fall out of the apple tree and be put on the compost heap. Neither of them got their wish. Dad, crippled by emphysema and stroke-induced dementia, became a lost-looking figure in a nursing home. Mum lived with me for five years before her death in 2009.

Mum's Alzheimer's was diagnosed in 1999. When she moved in with me I giggled with her when she talked about her 'brain not being big enough to hold all her memories'. Soon I was calming her when, at nightfall, she thought the world was ending. I held her as she sobbed that she wanted to die. I watched as her rational self fragmented.

But there were very few occasions when I felt she wasn't Mum. When I was angry with her it was Mum I was angry with, when I cried with her it was Mum I cried with. Two weeks before she died she looked straight at me, cupped my face in her hand and said 'You're a lovely person, sweetie-pie'. It was the first lucid sentence she'd uttered for months. It was *Mum* who uttered it. Her core self shone through until the day of her death.

I was asked to write about the carer's perspective on dementia, personhood and spirituality. I can't do that. Every carer is different. Each person with dementia is different. Each caring situation is different… Instead, I'll tell you about my perspective on Mum's dementia, about how Mum's dementia impacted on her personhood and on mine, and how our spirituality was affected by our joint battle with Mum's dementia.

THE DIAGNOSIS

The first I heard of it was when, during a telephone conversation, Mum's doctor uttered the words 'the diagnosis'. Eh? 'Which diagnosis?' I asked, my heart plummeting. Apparently my brother had been with Mum when she was diagnosed and had decided not to tell anyone. Mum hadn't mentioned it. I was furious. But as I expressed my fury I knew it was prompted by my being forced to face something I'd known for ages.

My weekly calls had become daily calls, then thrice-daily calls. 'She's getting frail,' I told myself, 'of course she needs cleaners, meals on wheels, reminders about appointments, etc.' The patching was all a desperate attempt to avoid the recognition that Mum's confusion was more than the normal effects of ageing.

Being told that a loved one has dementia is devastating. I imagine being told *you* have dementia is worse. Mum dealt with it by forgetting it. Very sensible, I thought. I was happy to go along with her, so the words 'dementia' and 'Alzheimer's' were never mentioned between us. I was open to her eventually wanting to talk about it but every time I purposely gave her an opening, she unerringly steered away from it. I didn't force it.

I assumed Mum would go into a care home. I visited a few near me. But only the specialist dementia homes would consider her. They frightened me. I couldn't do that to Mum. (I winced when I heard the government was encouraging earlier diagnosis: my priority would be making the diagnosis less disastrous, not making it earlier.)

So Mum came to live with me. We had always got on brilliantly, sharing a sense of humour, enthusiasm for life and endless curiosity. On the other hand, I'd always lived alone. I *liked* living alone. I also worked full time. It was daunting.

At first everything was easy. Mum's social competence was intact, and she had strategies to hide her appalling memory. Her self-confidence was good, and she was able to laugh at herself. Her story-telling ability was intact, as was her charm. She was straightforwardly good value.

She was soon made a mascot by my students, and my friends took her into their hearts. We were busy: dinners, lunches and teas, the cinema, theatre and opera; once, memorably, going to a garden party at Buckingham Palace. The Queen stopped six feet from Mum, who swooned with excitement. 'I *do* like living with you,' she would say.

But it couldn't last. Mum started to forget her stories. The end of a story would remind her of the beginning and she'd start again on an endless loop. She stopped telling stories. She 'read' books long after the story was lost to her. She suddenly lost interest. She read the newspaper but I had to censor it, removing all mention of suffering, war, famine or pestilence. The embroidery was next. She'd stitch all day, then, like Penelope in Homer's 'Odyssey', unpick it, berating herself for stupidity. I seemed to be threading a needle every ten seconds. I took it away. She didn't miss it. There was nothing left she could do by herself. But I couldn't be entertaining her all the time. She became lonelier and I became anguished.

NAVIGATING THE CARE SYSTEM

I had been resisting day care, thinking she would hate it. I was wrong. She blossomed: she adored the company, flirted with the men, talked nonsense to the women and charmed the staff. She would go off cheerfully in the morning and come back contentedly tired in the afternoon.

Mum started by going twice a week, but was soon going four times. I had some time to myself and got some work done. Mum and I had a break from each other. It was lovely to share worries with the staff and exchange banter with the drivers who collected her.

But soon Mum became incontinent. She wasn't sleeping well either. I was up several times at night, the washing machine was on constantly and I was run ragged. I dreaded Sunday and Monday, when I had her to entertain for a whole 48 hours. Work was relegated to the times when Mum dozed. Keeping Mum clean was getting difficult. She was tall and – er – robust. One night it took us an hour and a half to get her out of the bath. Mum was frightened of showers. Getting her to clean her teeth was a battle.

When Mum moved in I was told there was no point in my completing a carer's assessment. Social Services only became aware of my existence when Mum started day care. On completing my carer's assessment I discovered Mum was eligible for respite care. Six weeks a year! Bliss.

How wrong I was. I hugely enjoyed my first respite week and was looking forward to seeing Mum. But as the special transport bus drew up, Mum was looking out of the window. As she saw me her whole face collapsed. As she came down from the bus she was sobbing. She threw herself into my arms saying she wanted to die, that she was a bad person and that she was sorry. When I was able to get her coat off she was without a bra, her teeth had gone and she was covered in excrement. She also had the rash that told me her gluten-free diet (Mum was coeliac) had not been observed.

It took five weeks to stabilise her. I cancelled the other respite weeks. Other carers tell me they've had similar experiences. The five weeks were a nightmare. I took leave and devoted myself to Mum. She sobbed continually, wouldn't go to bed, looked petrified whenever she went near the bathroom and constantly said she wanted to die.

Mum had never been frightened of the dark but she was now. After being put to bed, she would get up every five minutes. I was screaming with exhaustion, worry and fear. Mum even became vicious. As I knelt to help her with her socks she intentionally kicked me in the face. She was constantly spiteful. It was all I could do not to respond in kind.

I lodged a formal complaint. The home fobbed me off. I persisted. But I dropped the complaint when I realised I was doing it only for the sake of others. For the first time in my life I wasn't prepared to go the extra mile. What use are formal complaint procedures if people haven't the energy to complete them?

Mum never fully recovered from this experience. She became needier and clingy. She would follow me around like a toddler. If I was out of sight for two seconds she'd come after me. She even followed me to the loo.

At about this point the special transport services changed their system. They warned us it might take a week or two to settle down. Four weeks later it was still a mess. They would collect Mum any time between eight and ten a.m. and drop her off any time between three and five p.m. Such a waste of my time. Dreadful to have to have Mum ready at eight, though they might not come until ten. Mum had no concept of time and couldn't understand what was going on. Neither could I.

So Social Services applied another plaster. Understandably they only give you something if you really, really need it, but this means that by the time you get it the next crisis is on the horizon. This plaster was direct payments. I was awarded £402 per week to buy in care so that I could continue working. I thought it would solve all my problems. It was the beginning of a whole new set.

I hired an agency. They promised a small team of experienced carers. The first week I counted 11 different people. Once I came home to find the carer with his coat on, bags piled at his feet, ready to go the minute I got home. The following day I was five minutes late. The carer had gone. I sacked the agency. This reduced my funding by 50 per cent. Social Services pay huge fees to incompetent agencies, but won't pay carers to do what agencies would otherwise do.

I had to advertise, field applications, conduct interviews, chase references, devise contracts, arrange for health and safety training and take out insurance. I discovered the joys of tax and national insurance, holiday pay, sick leave and the hollow feeling in your stomach when a carer thinks she's pregnant (and is therefore eligible for maternity leave).

I would come home from my full-time job only to allow a relieved carer to go home so that I could take over *her* job.

I once found myself staring at the Inland Revenue's website, tears streaming down my face, beside myself with anxiety. I have three degrees, am computer-literate and financially savvy; what on earth do others do, especially those carers who are themselves getting old and frail?

The final crisis came two months later. All my carers and their partners were part-time and worked shifts. My own timetable is far from set. Working out each weekly rota would take two or three hours. Then, doubtless, someone would be unable to do their stint and I'd have to start again.

One Sunday a carer told me she wasn't prepared to get Mum up any longer. Mum hated getting up. Her bad temper made it an unpleasant task. I couldn't blame the carer for not wanting to do it.

But it was the final straw. I started to sob and couldn't stop. Two hours later I was still sobbing. I was aware something had to be done. But I didn't know what to do. I would go to ring the doctor and then think 'no, he'll put her in a home'. I rang friends, but they were all out. Eventually I rang my lovely uncle and aunt. They drove down, called the doctor and that night took Mum back to Kent.

The wheels started turning to get Mum into a care home.

PERSONHOOD

A saving grace of Alzheimer's is that once firmly in its grip, people have no insight. Most of the time Mum lived with me she thought she was caring for me.

Before Mum came to live with me I read everything I could read about dementia. I spoke at length to Mum's consultant. I haunted the websites of organisations dealing with dementia and caring. Mum's consultant said that people rarely change personality, though it can seem that they are changing if they have been suppressing something.

I asked myself whether Mum had been suppressing anger, viciousness or manipulative tendencies. This made me smile. Mum was one of the most cheerful, optimistic and kind people I knew. This was hugely instrumental in enabling me to contemplate living with her.

Maybe what our consultant said is no longer received wisdom. But for us it was true. Mum's core self – her emotional self – survived the disintegration of her rational self.

Before Mum came to me I thought carefully about the things that made me *me*, and the things that made Mum *Mum*. Taking these to be 'non-negotiables', I brainstormed about how we might secure them for as long as possible.

For me this meant being able to work, socialise, exercise and get enough solitude. I saw that the last two would be the ones to go unless I was vigilant. One of the best decisions I made was that my bedroom and my study would be sacrosanct; places where Mum's paraphernalia and problems did not intrude. Throughout our years together I managed to exercise regularly by fiercely guarding my right to do this (and accepting every offer of help).

For Mum it meant autonomy, responsibility and socialising. I decided I would offer her as much choice as I could for as long as possible. I listed the jobs she would be able to do at different stages. I also decided I would integrate her into my own life as much as possible. This, I reasoned, would help because she wouldn't become an invisible hindrance, one I alone worried about, but rather a visible part of my life that everyone would have to recognise. I consciously decided that if this alienated anyone, so be it.

I also reflected on our respective strengths and weaknesses and how they might impact on our lives together. So I thought about Mum's infuriating (to me) habit of referring everything to herself and my infuriating (to her) habit of liking everything just so. I knew I'd have to do most of the changing, so I wrote out different strategies until I thought I had some that would work for both of us.

Looking back, I think this did work. As Mum's rational self fragmented, many aspects of her personality dissipated. But, if anything, Mum's dementia made her *more* of herself than she ever had been. It was as if her personality was distilled. All the unnecessary bits dropped away and Mum's essence was revealed.

Mum was energetic and driven. Despite having four children, she always worked. At first she was a secretary, but that frustrated her. So, at 40, despite having two children under five, she qualified as an international examiner in spoken English. At 70, in the year of her 50th wedding anniversary, she took a 2.1 in English Literature from Manchester University.

The dementia stopped Mum from *doing* things. Instead she had the time just to *be*. Despite taking after Mum in always having too much on, caring for her meant that I had to slow down too and just *be* with her. Together we gazed at the trails of the aeroplanes in the sky, we exclaimed at the neatness of bushes, at the beauty of silver cars and at the delightfulness of passing cats.

There were only three times during the time I cared for her that her personhood seemed to be slipping away.

The first was before she came to live with me. I went to see Mum often. Each time things were worse. She had given up housework, so the house was filthy. She had given up washing and changing, so she was filthy. There was nothing to eat in the house and the weight started to fall off her. Her eyes looked haunted and she began to look like a person with Alzheimer's. But when I took responsibility for hygiene, elegance and nutrition, all Mum had to do was sparkle. This she duly did.

The second time was before we started day care. I resisted it because I thought she'd hate it. But even if the rational Mum *would* have hated it, Mum was no longer her rational self, and she didn't hate it at all; she loved it.

The third time was before she went into a home. At this point I was in danger of losing *my* self too. I have heard talk of carers' dementia, and I think there is a great deal in the idea that the carer suffers as much from dementia as the cared for. I tried desperately to keep Mum out of a home. I worried myself sick about it. Again I was wrong. There comes a time when the only suitable companions for a person with dementia are other people with dementia. Professional care becomes a *sine qua non*. In resisting the home, I was again making the mistake of projecting Mum's rational self onto the person whose emotional self was now far more important.

Mum loved her care home. She adored music therapy, choral singing, dinner 'conversation' and the other activities. She teased the carers, and liked to dance or sing with them. She joined in cheerfully and wholeheartedly. When I visited her, her eyes lit up. She had no idea who I was but she 'knew I belonged to her' (as she once put it).

Once I saw she was settling, I relaxed and got my life back. I visited her often but I was no longer hands-on responsible for her care. It was liberating in the extreme. It was liberating for Mum too. When she had been with me, she had been watched every minute of every day. Poor Mum was never able so much as to get up without someone dancing attendance on her. Her nursing home was safe. She could wander the corridors at will, stare for hours out of the big picture windows and decide for herself when to go to bed. She had her autonomy back and she loved it.

It makes me feel guilty to know I had been inhibiting Mum's autonomy and her self-expression. I know she would know that I did it from love. But I still wish I hadn't done it. She should have gone into her nursing home six months before she did.

I believe the occasions when Mum's personality started to disintegrate had three things in common. The first is that in each case I had been projecting Mum's rational self into the decisions I'd been making. Mum's rational self used to be very strong. But that self had gone. The decisions I made on its basis were wrong. Whenever instead I made decisions in the light of Mum's emotional self, the decisions were right.

The recognition of this seems to me to make dementia less frightening. I know that if I get it (not unlikely, given both parents had it) the things that cause me *now* to curl up in horror won't be operative. Mum was a happy person before she had dementia, and she was a happy person afterwards. It is recognising *this*, not dwelling on what the earlier person would think if she could see herself now, that makes it possible to deal with dementia as it should be dealt with: practically.

The second was that something was stopping Mum from socialising. Mum's social side was extremely strong. It never left her. As she deteriorated I became responsible for her social life. Because I kept thinking Mum wouldn't want to socialise with others like her because she wouldn't want to think of herself as like them, I resisted things like day care and nursing homes. But Mum had gone past this point. She just wanted to be with people. And as soon as she found herself with people, she rallied. The fact that they were elderly and had dementia mattered not a jot. I was again projecting onto Mum my own fears.

Finally, the matter of autonomy is paramount. I had it right, I think, when I made Mum responsible for as much as possible when she came to live with me. If I were to run a nursing home I would make sure everyone did as much as possible for as long as possible – even if their 'help' means everything takes twice as long. In resisting Mum's going into a home – for the reasons outlined above – I was maintaining a situation in which her autonomy was compromised. Once she was in a safe environment, and could make her own decisions, she came into her own again.

SPIRITUALITY

Mum became a Christian in her forties. It might have been a reaction to Dad's atheism. She embraced it with vigour: running the Parochial Church Council, singing in the choir, reading the lesson and teaching in Sunday school. Despite protests, my brother and I were required to go to church with her every Sunday.

She was an intellectual Christian. She studied her Bible and asked herself what it all meant. But she was not a pushover. If she didn't like the things she heard she would find some way to make sense of other people believing them. She didn't feel she had to believe them herself.

I adopted my father's atheism. I thought the whole thing Christian thing was a nonsense. Mum and I would argue for hours about Christianity, the church and the point of it all. To her credit she never once said, though she must have thought, you'll be more understanding when you grow up.

If she did think this, she was right. In my forties I too became a believer as a result of attempting to show that human beings are nothing more than sophisticated computers. I thought the objections to this view would be easily overcome. Once again I was wrong.

The objections proved so intractable that I began to think – I want to say 'to *see*' – that human beings are far more than computers. For the first time ever I began to appreciate the importance of our capacity to value things, of the fact that things *matter* to us. I also took on board properly our ability to assign *meaning*. I began to think that such things could be explained only by appeal to God.

Forty years of thinking atheism is the only rational position isn't an easy view to dislodge, but in the end I had to admit to myself that I was no longer an atheist, nor even an agnostic, but a fully fledged believer.

Culturally, of course, I was a Christian. I worshipped at church because of this. I enjoyed the familiarity. But I couldn't believe, despite trying very hard, in Christ's divinity. At first it bothered me. I spent several years trying out other religions, but I didn't find any that suited. In the end I decided it wouldn't bother God if I worshipped in church, so it shouldn't bother me either.

People often ask whether my belief was instrumental in bringing Mum to live with me. It is difficult to answer this. I brought Mum to live with me because I loved her and couldn't have put her in any of the care homes I saw at the time. I believe that God IS love, and throughout the time Mum lived with me I felt very strongly that I was doing the right thing. But I find it difficult to believe that my atheist self wouldn't have acted precisely as my believing self did.

My faith did, however, support me through some of the worse times. I felt God was present throughout, not just for me but for Mum too, and that was very comforting.

Before Mum came to live with me, her church was wonderful. Someone rang her every week to see if she wanted a lift. They collected her for choir practice. They did everything they could to involve her in the life of the church. At this time I was chairing the National Forum for Values in Education and the Community, and in charge of promoting the spiritual, moral, social and cultural development of pupils aged five to nineteen. This was in the wake of the Bulger murder and there was a sense that we were all going to hell in a hand-cart.

But as I travelled around the country discussing this, I was hugely aware that in one corner of our country at least, things were absolutely as they should be. One small parish church was making one confused old lady, battling with the beginnings of dementia, feel that she was an important part of their community. It was humbling.

When Mum came to me we started by going to church every Sunday. The church was a pleasant five minutes' walk from the house. Mum was more than capable of this, and she loved the familiar hymns and prayers. She also enjoyed the socialising afterwards.

But then the walk started to become painful. Mum would ask every ten seconds, 'Where are we going?' 'To church,' I would reply. 'Why?' she would say. Her faith didn't seem to mean anything to her any more.

I asked the vicar if he thought someone might be able to give us a lift (at that time I didn't drive). But I heard nothing. I put a notice up in the church hall asking if anyone could help us. No one replied. We stopped going. No one ever got in touch to ask why. I still haven't forgiven them.

But music, and in particular hymns and carols, were a major source of meaning for Mum. You might be interested in an extract from my blog,[1] written just before Mum's final Christmas:

> The evening didn't start well. Some students were coming to sing carols. So everyone was walked or wheeled into one of the sitting rooms. With about 50 residents, staff, relatives and a lot of wheelchairs, it was a bit of a squeeze.
>
> The students arrived and walked self-consciously into the space left for them. They launched into 'Hark the herald angels sing'.
>
> Mum was electrified. Slowly she got up and moved towards the choir. I considered stopping her but she wasn't doing any harm so I followed. She walked into their midst and stood transfixed with wonder. At the end of the carol, she looked at them, then at me, then at them again. Then she said, 'Oh, I love you, I love you, I love you all.'
>
> When they resumed Mum sang along with them. She couldn't remember the words of course. But she had the tune bang on. And her voice is still lovely. As is her smile! Toothless, but so expressive of love and pleasure that I felt quite tearful. I doubt the choristers will ever feel as appreciated as they did that night. My heart almost burst with love and pride.

I completely agree with those who say that music is the way to reach people with dementia. Spiritual music – hymns and carols – especially so, if the person has been familiar with them in earlier life: everything else may be long gone, but the tunes remain.

AFTERTHOUGHTS

Mum died in April 2009. It was very sudden. The last night was bad, but no worse than childbirth. I was with her throughout and holding her hand as she died. I had just about got used to her being in a home.

It is now a year since her death and I have had time to assimilate it and reflect on what the years of caring mean to me.

It was not clear to me, when I took Mum on, that I would be any good at caring for someone. I am not a natural carer. I was intrigued to see how I would manage. I surprised myself. I found a patience I would never have predicted. I also found a joy in caring for Mum that I could never have found in any other way. Having to slow down to her pace of life was very therapeutic and made me aware of the downside of the frenetic pace of my usual life. Looking at life through Mum's eyes brought into focus all sorts of things I would never otherwise have noticed.

Becoming a carer also revealed to me something that otherwise would have remained invisible: the world of caring. There is a whole section of our society that remains below the radar of 'normal' people: the thousands who devote their lives to the care of others. These people are not saints; they are funny, furious, feisty and, when crossed, fearsome. But they live in a parallel universe.

In recent years, the world of caring has started to become more visible. The expected explosion of dementia is likely to increase its visibility. I do hope so. In a world in which designer shoes, celebrity shenanigans and bankers' bonuses are everyday news, the recognition that so many people put love first is, in my opinion, such an important corrective.

NOTE

1. Marianne's blog 'Keeping Mum', written for Saga Magazine Online, will be published as a book by Hay House in 2011.

CHAPTER 4

Walking with a Person into Dementia

Creating Care Together

Elizabeth MacKinlay

INTRODUCTION: THE EXPERIENCE OF DEMENTIA

Dementia is still a feared condition and perhaps fear is one of the greatest barriers to quality life for those who have dementia. Too often people with dementia are shut off from others in the community and may even be isolated within and from their own families. It was this factor that really struck me when I began working with Christine Bryden soon after her initial diagnosis. Christine and I first met more than a decade ago. We were both members of a Christian group on a Cursillo[1] team in 1995, preparing for a forthcoming Cursillo. It was during those weeks of preparation that her diagnosis of early onset Alzheimer's disease was confirmed, following extensive investigations and involving a second medical opinion. This was the beginning of a devastating time for Christine and a shock for the rest of us who were her friends and working on the Cursillo team with her. It was hard to believe that someone so capable and high achieving in all that she did, was suddenly getting lost on the way home from work.

At our final session of Cursillo, Christine invited me to walk the journey into dementia with her as her spiritual director (spiritual guide). Her invitation came, she said, because I was both a geriatric nurse and a priest; she felt she needed both. This journey was to become a major learning experience for me.

THE IMPACT OF DIAGNOSIS

People with early onset of dementia, such as Christine, are often in the middle of a career and may still have young children and financial commitments. All of these roles and expectations are suddenly shaken as they struggle to come to terms with the diagnosis of Alzheimer's disease. 'Devastating' is an expression used by some people newly diagnosed. None of us can easily come to terms with such a diagnosis; it takes time and special love and care. Later in the progress of her disease, Christine's dementia was re-diagnosed as fronto-temporal dementia, which is not uncommon in cases of early onset dementia.

Christine had only been a Christian for a few years when she received her diagnosis of dementia. Her faith provided a strong focus for hope in the midst of her world view, including her roles in life, that seemed to be about to disintegrate. Christine spoke of experiencing an awful fear of ceasing to be; this seems to be present for a lot of relatives and friends too, who think that as the dementia increases the person will not be there any more, or that they will become merely an empty shell. While this view has been prevalent, authors such as Kitwood (1997a), Goldsmith (1996, 2004) and Hughes, Louw and Sabat (2006) dispute it and present alternatives that affirm the continuing of the person, despite communication difficulties.

Christine's relationship with God was the one thing that was sustaining her in the midst of coming to terms with the diagnosis, the depression and all the things that were happening for her at that time. As she struggled with these factors that went to the core of who she was, this question of 'would she lose God?' became a crucial one for her. From the Christian perspective, God would still be there, but the other question, 'would she still have a sense of God being there?', was a different matter. In the intervening years Christine has come to realize that, even when the cognitive structure and some of the emotional overlays disappear, right at the centre of one's being is the spiritual. Thus she is still loved by God and still held by God at the centre. I think this process has become so much more profound for her with the passage of time. Perhaps even writing her second book has helped her to articulate the nature of that continuing relationship with God (Bryden 2005). At one point Christine said that having a limited time frame on her life, becoming aware of the fact that her condition would lead to death, made her more intentional about seeking to deepen her relationship with God.

The spiritual dimension does not need cognitive structure and language for expression; it is situated more deeply within what it means to be human.

WHAT IS SPIRITUALITY?

The spiritual domain is worked out through life meaning and it is mediated through relationship with others and/or a deity, through the environment and all creation, through the arts and, for many people, through religious practices. For many others, although there is no practice of religion, the spiritual is worked out through experiences of relationship with others, through the wonder of nature and music, art, drama. The spiritual is related to the sense of awe that is felt in deep relationship, or in seeing a beautiful sunrise, or experiencing music or art at a very deep level.

LIFE MEANING AND DEMENTIA

If dementia can be talked about and the meaning of that diagnosis shared with others in a trusting relationship, the person with dementia may be greatly helped. If it is possible to see meaning and accept that, this opens the way to hope and wellbeing. This is a matter of the spiritual domain.

A SPIRITUAL PROCESS FOR FINDING LIFE MEANING (A PROCESS OF SPIRITUAL TASKS)

It is from our hearts that we find hope and can reach out to friends and family. An important part of this spiritual process is a journey with someone in a trusting relationship, to explore meaning. We can use a process called spiritual reminiscence to explore meaning, either in small groups of people or on a one-to-one basis with a spiritual guide or partner.

SPIRITUAL JOURNEY WITH A PERSON WITH DEMENTIA

Spiritual direction, in the Christian tradition, is accompanying someone over a period of time, supporting, reflecting and engaging with them on the life journey. To journey together, one person walks with the other and helps them to reflect on their life and to deepen their spiritual journey and to find meaning in the process of their life experiences. In the Christian context, it involves developing a deepening relationship with God, through Christ. It was both a challenge and a privilege to begin this journey with Christine. A challenge, because I did not know whether this relationship of spiritual guide with someone who had dementia would work, and a privilege, as I was walking on holy ground; I was beginning an unknown journey. This was an unknown journey because, although I had been a spiritual guide before, I had always worked with people who had their cognitive abilities.

My knowledge base as a nurse led me initially to ask myself questions such as 'how can I effectively do spiritual direction with a person who has a diagnosis of dementia?' By definition, a person with dementia has problems with communicating and memory. How can spiritual direction or spiritual reminiscence be used in such instances?

DEMENTIA AS A TOPIC OF CONVERSATION

When I began working with Christine in the mid-1990s, I found that for the first time in my professional career as a nurse I was challenged to meet with her as a person first, and as someone with dementia second. Nurses have traditionally learned how to 'manage' dementia, although that is changing as person-centred care is becoming more widely accepted and practised. Based on my experience of journeying with Christine, and subsequent research with other people who have dementia, I contend now that dementia should not be managed; the best management can leave the person isolated in the middle of this disease. A motif of journey seems to provide the best way of being and working with these people, always engaging with them as care-partners on the journey, where both the person with dementia and fellow travellers on the journey are active in person-centred care.

With Christine I was able to talk freely about dementia; we named it, and we focused on the meaning of it for her. Christine was the centre of our conversations. I was learning how to do this too. I found that it was more important to be a person journeying with her, as a care-partner, not an expert. The role that fitted best was pastoral care. This was the beginning of an intentional friendship with Christine.

Christine had been told by her doctor that she could expect to be in a nursing home within five years (Boden[2] 1998). It is hard to fight against such predictions. Early in our meetings Christine talked about the fear of losing her 'self' as she moved deeper into dementia.

She shared her perception of the sudden crisis of identity: the day before her diagnosis her identity included being a successful single mother and working at a high level in the public service, and the next day she was simply being labelled as a person with dementia. She said, 'My world had collapsed, everything had changed, I faced a defeat of spirit and hope' (verbal communication). Fear was part of this journey, particularly in the early stages.

Thus we began this journey of spiritual direction and guidance. In the spiritual direction sessions we talked about her day-to-day life in her walk into dementia. We talked about whatever was on her mind at that time. She spoke of her children and their family relationships, of not being able to work and the financial implications of that. These conversations were part of our journeying in the process of spiritual direction. I note here that while I listened to her concerns about financial matters, my role there was not to solve these, as that lay outside of my spiritual guide role, but I certainly listened.

The questions about God kept coming up again and again; her faith journey was vitally important to her. My most important role in this journey was to listen and to reflect back to her issues that she raised, helping her to clarify and to go deeper in her reflections. Another important topic for her was how she could and would speak to her three daughters about having dementia. In fact, she involved her daughters right from the beginning, and each one of them responded according to her own personality and her own level of maturity and ability to understand.

Christine expressed some concerns, for example, about not being able to pray spontaneously, as she had been able to before the onset of her dementia; the words would not come. We talked about this problem and decided that she would try to use set prayers from a book of prayers that she could read in her daily quiet time. This worked for her, in providing her with support when she could not find the words herself. Depression occurs not uncommonly with dementia and is another part that is hard to deal with. I remember Christine being quite depressed in the early months after her diagnosis. She spoke about a sense of blackness that she experienced, of not being able to move, or do anything, just being there in the dark. Then she found that she wasn't alone in the dark. God was there with her, and she realized that she could draw some strength and some hope in the midst of this dreadful experience. It was when her depression lifted that she was able to pray more easily again.

As we continued to meet regularly, I realized that what we spoke of was too important not to be shared with others. I was learning that it was possible to work spiritually with someone who has dementia. Indeed, Christine responded very well to the conversations that we had. So I suggested that Christine should write down her experiences and what we had talked about each week. I suggested that it might be possible to write a book that would be very helpful for others experiencing dementia and for their care-partners. In some ways, it was easier for her to write than to find the right words while speaking. She has come an enormous distance since that time, in both her faith journey and her understanding of what it means to live as a person with dementia.

Christine has been travelling this journey since 1995. In her second book (Bryden 2005) her focus changed: now she was writing not about 'Who will I be?' but 'Who I am becoming?'. Christine wrote that, underneath the outer confusion, the true self remains intact despite the ravages of dementia.

It was her description of these changes that touched me deeply, being aware of the spiritual journey that had continued to evolve over the years since I had first met her. Now, having written not just one book, but two, Christine reflected on her spiritual journey and dementia and she wrote:

> For me, dementia is a journey to a spiritual self. I have learnt how to dance with dementia, how to adapt to change, how to express my needs, and how to stay in tune with the music as it slows. (Bryden and MacKinlay 2008, p.135)

Christine then spoke about her spiritual self that exists in the 'now' without necessarily acknowledging a past or a future, but living in the present. She is suggesting that the essence of being human is what lies at the core of our being.

As we continued to meet over the weeks and months, I found that I was learning so much that was right outside the traditional understandings of Western medicine, which defines the person with dementia as the disease rather than as a person. I was seeing Christine as an individual in her context and I was coming to know her at a deeper level.

In her second book Christine has written of 'dancing with dementia'; this image speaks of her changing relationship with her husband as her primary care-partner, and with herself, with dementia, as they continue this journey together as care-partners (Bryden 2005). The image of dancing with dementia formed a powerful picture of continuing relationship changes, coupled with continual adjustments to each other's needs as the disease progressed. In this perspective, caring is not 'doing' for the other person who can't do for themselves any longer, so much as asking, 'What is it that you need from me and what is it that I need from you?' This care-partnership can become a valuable model.

In a rather wonderful way, in the midst of the decline that is happening to Christine now, including the difficulties she has sometimes with her cognitive abilities, the spiritual part is still there. The journey with Christine has raised questions about what is ultimately important in life. Too often we judge people by what they do in life and their positions in society, rather than looking at the person themselves and the depth of their being. But for me the part which was critical and most wonderful in Christine's second book was that journey into the divine, if you like, that moving into the spiritual and into the depths of one's being (Bryden 2005).

THE COMPLEXITIES OF COMMUNICATING WITH A PERSON WHO HAS DEMENTIA

Often, after a diagnosis of dementia, the family and the person who has dementia find it very difficult to talk about what the person is experiencing. It may well be the beginning of two parallel conversations; conversations between the family members and health providers, and conversations of the person with dementia, perhaps with the health care providers. This means that the person with dementia may discover that it is impossible to find anyone they can speak openly with. In the worst cases, there is no one to listen to the fears, hopes and concerns of the person living with dementia. Finding the right words in a timely manner can prove too hard for the person with dementia who is struggling with communication.

When my mother was in residential aged care with dementia, a commonly asked question to me was, 'Does she know who you are?' To me this was the wrong question. How can I know if she knows who I am? This is not about a test of my mother's cognitive abilities. My mother is my mother, even if our relationship has changed. In the difficulties of communication within this disease, what matters more is how I reach out to communicate with my mother, or others with dementia.

Christine's comment, 'I know that I know you, but not why I know you' (Bryden 2005, p.110) takes us into the complexity of the communication processes of dementia. At one point, Christine said that although she may forget the person's name, she still 'knows who you are'. Christine has lost some of her ability to process names and persons, but there is more to knowing than connecting the correct name with the face. It could be said that Christine has recognized that she knows, but the specific label seems to have been lost. The sense of knowing goes more deeply than just putting a label or a name on the outside, and that is something I've been very aware of with Christine.

Some of the work of Damasio (2003) in neurobiology may help explain what is happening for Christine and others who have dementia. Current tests of cognitive function still leave much to be explained about the thoughts, understanding and behaviour of people who live with dementia. According to Damasio, emotions and feelings have complex origins and, applying his theories, it is likely that aspects of neurobiological functioning are still present and may explain Christine's sense of 'knowing'. Recognising her communication problems, Christine remarked: 'I need many more clues to help me tune into your recollections of events, and many helpful hints as to who you are, so that somewhere along the way I can gain a glimpse of my own shattered memories.' Christine is developing strategies to deal with her changing cognitive structure to help her to make connections. She said: 'I am slowly learning how to live without remembering labels: your name, or even my name. I know faces and know I connect with them somehow, but not why I know them and what I know about them' (Bryden and MacKinlay 2008, pp.143–144).

DOES SPIRITUAL REMINISCENCE WORK WITH YOUNGER PEOPLE?

Generally spiritual reminiscence is less relevant to younger people, because often younger people have not begun to think about the deeper things of life and to reflect on the meaning and purpose of their lives. But for younger people with dementia, like Christine, it can work because with their diagnosis these people face a crisis of identity and meaning in life. Spiritual reminiscence is a way into dealing with these very issues that are central to the wellbeing of younger people with dementia. In spiritual reminiscence and spiritual care and direction, it is possible at least to share the burden one-on-one with another person who will simply listen, and not judge or tell the person what to do. A sense of trust and openness and love is essential. Being open to possibilities and hope at all times is essential.

The trust that can be facilitated through spiritual care is the basis for spiritual growth and opening to new ways of being, when living with dementia. This changes the focus to being able to ask, 'What can I do and be?', rather than 'What can't I do and be?' Using a spiritual approach can help the person affirm their identity again, in this new place of living with dementia. It can go to the core of their being, to strip away the things that are not important, to focus on what is important. The process of spiritual reminiscence always respects and supports the person with dementia. It assists by affirming who they are in this journey, allowing them to share their deepest fears and hopes. It provides a safe place just to 'be'.

Dementia is a progressive disease, albeit for most a slowly progressing condition. The needs for spiritual support vary throughout this journey. More recently, Christine described her experience of dementia as 'I'm like the swan, gliding above the water, paddling frantically beneath the surface,' in order to keep up with life.

Christine continues to need the love and support of others in her daily journey. She needs to continue to have people with whom she can share her concerns and her feelings. She needs to be listened to and affirmed as a person of worth, simply as being made in the image of God.

ARE THERE OTHERS LIKE CHRISTINE, WHO CAN RESPOND TO SPIRITUAL SUPPORT AND GUIDANCE?

As I had journeyed so closely with Christine, I needed to ask if what I was seeing with her, and her ability to continue to function emotionally and spiritually, were unique to Christine. Could it be the same for other people who have dementia? I had to ask, does Christine do so well because she had a high level of intelligence when she was diagnosed? Would other people with dementia respond in similar ways, if they had the opportunity to share with others in a supported environment? Would Christine just prove to be an exceptional person, even with dementia? We needed evidence to see if what I had learnt in journeying with Christine might be the same for others too. This led to seeking and obtaining research grants to examine the experience of dementia and where people with dementia find meaning in life (MacKinlay, Trevitt and Coady 2002–2005; MacKinlay, Trevitt and Hobart 2002; Trevitt and MacKinlay 2004, 2006). We continue to study ways of communicating more effectively with people who have dementia. We are trialling programs that may be used to lighten depression among people with dementia.

THE PLACE OF FAITH IN CHRISTINE'S EXPERIENCE OF DEMENTIA

It was Christine's faith that first brought us together on this journey into dementia. Through this last decade, it has been her faith that has sustained her. As it becomes increasingly difficult for her to communicate, it will be her community of faith that will support her. This disease clearly illustrates the interdependency of human beings. While much emphasis is placed on autonomy and self-sufficiency, dementia strips these protective outer shields away, and each person with dementia is left vulnerable in a community that values independence, not interdependence. A great strength of Christianity is the community that it makes possible, worked out through the body of Christ, which is the term used to describe the community that is made up of each congregation or group of believers. We all have need of each other, and people with dementia can teach those who do not have dementia what it means to live in the moment, and be inspirational in their striving for connection with others.

From a faith perspective dementia also provides the opportunity to connect deeply one with another, until late in the disease. At that point, the community of faith becomes the memory, the supporter and nourisher of the person with dementia. Christine recognized the importance of this support from her community of faith when she said: 'As I travel towards the dissolution of myself, my personality, my very essence, my relationship with God needs increasing support from you' (Bryden and MacKinlay 2002, p.74). She's talking in a Christian sense here, and says, 'Don't abandon me at any stage, for the Holy Spirit connects us, it links our souls, our spirits, not our minds or brains. I need you to minister to me, to sing with me, pray with me, to be my memory for me' (p.74). The essence of her belief is the connection between people at the deepest spiritual level, spirit to spirit, where the person with dementia is nourished and supported by the spirituality of the caring community. For her as a Christian, the Holy Spirit is the presence of God within each one of us, bringing us close together in spiritual fellowship.

The journey into dementia is a complex and tortuous one. Dementia is so widely feared that the mere knowledge of the diagnosis can isolate people from each other. The disease affects not only the person diagnosed, but their family and close friends. Often friends and even family may stop being with, or visiting, the person who has dementia as the disease progresses. Yet, as Christine so clearly shows, it is possible to communicate and connect with people who have dementia. We must not allow the disease to get in the way of that communication.

NOTES

1. 'Cursillo' is the term used for a short intensive course in Christian faith and spiritual growth and development.
2. First book published as Christine Boden, the second as Christine Bryden, after her marriage.

ACKNOWLEDGMENT

Christine Bryden has been consulted throughout the writing of the chapter and is in full agreement to its publication.

CHAPTER 5

Becoming a Friend of Time

A Consideration of how we may Approach Persons with Dementia through Spiritual Sharing in the Moment

John Killick

Mindfulness is an approach to human experience that is making inroads into Western thought and practice. Perhaps its essence is encapsulated in the following quotations from a Vietnamese Zen Master, Thich Nhat Hanh:

> Our true home is in the present moment. To live in the present moment is a miracle.

> Attentive to each moment, my mind is clear like a calm river.

> We need only to bring our body and mind into the present moment, and we will touch what is refreshing and healing and wondrous.

> (2009)

Books by Hanh and other Buddhist teachers are approaching best-seller status in America and the UK. Dismissed by some as 'alternative religion' on a par with 'alternative medicine', adherents are convinced that we have much to learn from breaking down the barriers erected by traditional theism.

A parallel, and even more surprising development has been that of 'positive psychology'. This was founded by Martin Seligman in the United States, who perceived that conventional reactive approaches, concentrating on developing techniques for coping with mental illness, were missing half the story. He defines the movement as follows: 'a psychology of positive human functioning…that achieves a scientific understanding and effective interventions to build thriving individuals, families and communities' (Seligman 2005, p.7).

Research into aspects of positive psychology has taken a number of innovative turns, and one of these is 'mindfulness'. Jon Kabat-Zinn describes it as: 'being in the moment with things exactly as they are, without trying to change anything' (2005, p.20).

I begin with these observations because I shall be attempting to draw a parallel with the views of some individuals, either with dementia or familiar with people with dementia, about a noteworthy aspect of the condition, which may be significant in any discussion of spirituality in this context. Before proceeding to that discussion, however, I shall provide some quotations, and some more extended examples from my own and others' experience.

By way of introduction to the quotations I feel it is important to draw a distinction between the physical and psychosocial aspects of dementia. No description of how the person presents, both to him or herself and to others, can possibly be complete if it is confined to medical characteristics. Though many physical illnesses have a psychological component, dementia is unusual in the degree to which the progress of the condition is dependent upon wellbeing. Tom Kitwood was probably the first psychologist in Britain to highlight the crucial relevance of the way a person with dementia is treated, and encouraged to see themselves, for the development of characteristics of the condition. In copious writings, culminating in the seminal text *Dementia Reconsidered* (1997a), he enumerated the damaging effects of negative attitudes and promoted the ideal of coming alongside the person to understand, share and encourage. He even posited the concept of 'rementia' in those who were to be offered a social environment wholly favourable to the preservation of their personhood.

An understanding of how time may be experienced by persons with dementia is central to the process of empathising with them. Because dementia has serious consequences for the capacity to remember, cutting off access to short-term memories and often damaging the reasoning capacity, it is clear that the notion of subjectivity may be changed. It is through our memories that we evaluate the past, and without this bedrock we would be unable to imagine what might come next, and the consequences of our actions. Lacking this pattern-making capacity, we would lose the sense of continuity that is essential to those of us living busy and demanding lives.

Various authors have described the consequences for the person of this fundamental change in perception. The Canadian novelist and politician Michael Ignatieff, whose mother had dementia, expressed it as follows:

> People with dementia are not vegetables, but primary selves. They are no longer like us, busy and full of purpose, bent on becoming something.

> Instead they are prisoners of the realm of pure being. In this realm there is only now, this instant. (Ignatieff 1992)

Another Canadian, Debbie Everett, is a hospital chaplain who has worked extensively with people with dementia; she sums up what she has learned in the following words:

> For those of us who are cognitively intact, time is like a stream of water in which we float with the current. For someone with Alzheimer's Disease time is frozen into individual snowflakes that touch the skin and melt. (Everett 1996, p.85)

Lisa Snyder is a social worker in America who has edited a valuable compilation of narratives by people with dementia; here is a key description:

> For Bill the past is elusive and the future uncertain. A relationship with him can be demanding – but also deeply inspiring. Like a Zen Master he exacts my conscious attention to each present moment and renews my appreciation for the unpredictable and spontaneous dimensions of life. (Snyder 2002, p.56)

The comparison with a Zen Master chimes with the introductory paragraphs of this chapter.

People with dementia have also pinpointed in their writings the change in perception of time as a significant consequence of dementia. Christine Bryden, an Australian, has written two books since receiving the diagnosis. In the second of these occurs the following passage:

> I am more stretched out somehow, more linear, more step-by-step in my thoughts. I have lost the vibrancy, the buzz of interconnectedness, the excitement and focus I once had. I have lost the passion, the drive that once characterised me. I am like a slow-motion version of my old self – not physically but mentally. (Bryden 2005, pp.101–102)

Cary Smith Henderson, an American with dementia, in his book *Partial View* (Henderson and Andrews 1998), prints one of his poems, of which this is a part:

> Every day
> Is a new day.
> I've never seen
> This day before
> And chances are
> I'll never see it again.
> Every day is separate.

You don't know
What's going to happen
In any one day.
It's as if every day
You have never seen
Anything before
Like what you're seeing right now.
Every day is absolutely separate
And every minute is separate.
No two minutes are anywhere near alike…

(p.41)

Elsewhere Henderson gives an account of what this focusing down can mean:

I will pick up leaves, probably the same as I had before. I love the fall colours. I pick 'em up anyhow, whether I have them or not. Every year it seems like they're prettier and prettier. I appreciate them a lot more now than I did a few years ago. When I can't do the big things I can do the little things. Things are a lot more precious than they were. I go ape on the leaves. (p.77)

There now follow two extended descriptions of interactions, each of which lasted about seven minutes, and both of which concentrate on the moment and the riches it may contain. One involves myself (based on the film *When Your Heart Wants to Remember* (BBC/RCN 1999[1])), and the other a well-known therapist, based on the DVD *There is a Bridge* (TMK Productions and Memory Bridge 2007[2]). Being filmed, these permit analysis in some detail, without relying upon the memory of the two instigators. As I was a participant in the first, however, my own feelings and interpretations necessarily play a part. In the second, the therapist's comments on the process are interwoven:

1. BRONWEN

I was visiting the nursing home for the first time, and a film crew was recording my first half-hour in the dementia unit. The first person I encountered was Bronwen (a member of staff whispered her name to me). She was sitting in a corridor, so I knelt down in an attempt to engage her in eye contact; this was unsuccessful, as she persisted in looking beyond me over my shoulder. After introducing myself I asked her if she would like to have a chat; there was no reply. (I had no idea at this stage whether

Bronwen had any verbal language left.) I passed a few inconsequential remarks without gaining any response, and excused myself and moved on into the lounge area.

Here I had a couple of somewhat desultory conversations with residents, before the door opened and Bronwen entered; she had a resolute expression on her face and was clearly looking for me. I held my hands out to her and she took them. Somebody, possibly the film director, said 'Nice tie.' (I was wearing a particularly vivid tie with an uncomplicated design which I had found elicited positive responses on previous occasions.) I said to Bronwen, 'Do you like the tie? You can touch it,' and I held it out to her. Bronwen ran her fingers from bottom to top of the tie whilst studying it, then turned away. I took her hands again. She pointed towards a table and chairs. 'Would you like to sit down?' I asked. She nodded and said, 'Yes.'

I brought her over to the table and helped her to a seat at one end. 'May I sit here?' I asked, indicating a chair next to her. Again she nodded and said, 'Yes.' I pulled the chair up close, then, holding both of her hands, stared into her eyes. This time she did not look away. 'It's good to see you. You can say what you like.' At this last remark she gave a little shudder, which in retrospect I have interpreted as a slightly dismayed reaction, as if she realised that I hadn't yet understood the nature of the interaction.

She commenced a movement with her left hand clasped in my right, which at first I interpreted as a shaking of hands, a physical greeting, but then increased in speed and intensity: it had turned into a game, quite a vigorous one, until it eventually spent itself.

Bronwen pointed into the distance and I guessed she was indicating a vase of flowers further down the table. As I brought the vase towards her I said, 'These flowers, aren't they beautiful!' She raised a finger to her lips with a very quiet 'shh', so I did the same, acknowledging that words were to play a minor part in this conversation.

Bronwen reached out and touched the blooms. Her fingers were wet, so she wiped them on the wooden arm of her chair. There followed a comprehensive exploration of the properties of the chair-arm, and this discovery extended to my hand, which was resting there. She then transferred her hand to my inner thigh, but since she was employing the back of her hand for this purpose I believe she was examining the texture of my trousers, and that this action lacked any sexual content.

While she carried out this sensory activity she did not once look down, but we maintained an intense mutual gaze. Then she looked around at the film crew. The expression on her face did not seem to indicate puzzlement at their presence, rather she was looking at them out of contentment with her relationship. When she looked away from me I did not alter my gaze, so that when she looked back at my face she saw that I was still there for her.

Bronwen pointed again; this time it was past the vase of flowers and she seemed to be indicating something outside the window. She nodded and said 'Yes' again, and I mirrored her exactly. I had no idea what she was looking at, but it didn't seem to matter − I was caught in the web of our togetherness. Then she seemed distracted momentarily by the crew, so I gently touched her on the shoulder to recall her to the inner circle created by our arms and gaze. She began running her hand over the chair-arm again, so I replaced my hand there and she caressed it.

By this time we were both getting tired, and it showed in her face and gestures particularly. Bronwen gently placed my hands together on the table-top, nodded, said 'Yes,' and lay back in her chair. I followed suit. She appeared so exhausted that I did not expect any further communication from her, but she pulled herself upward again in a last effort; this time she did not speak but nodded deeply. Her eyes were closed, but when her head rested again on the chair-back she uttered the word 'wonderful'.

I asked staff afterwards about Bronwen's speech, and they told me that although she had been in the home for four months, the only words she had been heard to utter were 'yes' and 'no'.

2. GLADYS

Gladys is a woman aged 87 years with Alzheimer's, and in this description she is interacting with the well-known communicator and founder of Validation Therapy, Naomi Feil.

At the outset Gladys is seen sitting in a chair with her eyes almost closed, slowly tapping her hand on the arm of the chair and moving her legs back and forward slightly. She appears disengaged from her surroundings, living in her own separate world. On encountering such a person, many would doubt whether anything meaningful was going on in Gladys's mind and whether any communication was possible. Naomi comments: 'When people are very old and deteriorated and no-one enters their world and they're just sitting there, they will withdraw inward more and more, and their desperate need for connection is all now inside.'

Naomi begins by approaching Gladys from the front and asking her, 'Mrs W, hello! Do you want me to sit? Can you see me good?' Gladys reaches up and pushes Naomi's shoulder in the direction of the chair, so Naomi sits. Gladys holds Naomi's hand and moves it in a rhythmical way. (Naomi describes this as belonging to 'the phase of repetitive motion'.) Gladys has a tear on her cheek, and Naomi draws attention to this, commenting that she seems to have pain in her face and that she looks sad. She asks, 'Is it scary? Are you afraid?' and begins to massage Gladys's cheekbones. She comments that this 'is where the mother usually touches the child... Every cell remembers where it was touched by the mother, and often that person knows, even if they can't say a word.'

Now Naomi ventures, 'Can you let me in a little bit, do you think, just a little?' Eye contact is strongly held, and Gladys beats her hand on the arm of her chair. Naomi continues, 'Maybe I could be with you and Jesus for a minute?' This leads into the first singing episode. Naomi sings 'Jesus loves me, this I know, for the Bible tells me so', and matches the force and pace of her singing with Gladys's movements on the chair-arm, and sometimes on Naomi's shoulder. Naomi explains: 'I use music because when speech is gone, especially with Gladys...it was religious music, there's emotion and safety tied to it. What I did was, when she moved, I moved with her, and when I was singing (for she didn't sing with me) I matched the intensity of her movement, and pretty soon, for a split second, we became one person.'

The next stage is described by Naomi as follows: 'At one point, when she got very quiet and very peaceful, and my voice became very quiet and very peaceful, and my breathing slowed to her breathing, she pulled me to her, and I moved with her, and I believe at that moment I was a symbol of her Mom.'

'Can you open your eyes now? Can you sing with me?' asks Naomi. She begins to sing, whilst continuing to stroke Gladys's cheeks: 'He's got the whole world in his hands...'. When she reaches the second verse Gladys joins in with 'in his hands' three times, and then with the whole of the last line, 'He's got the whole world in his hands'. Finally Naomi asks, 'Do you feel safe?' 'Yes,' Gladys answers. 'Do you feel safe with Jesus?' 'Yes.' 'And me?' Gladys nods.

Naomi comments: 'The breakthrough doesn't happen every time, the person doesn't always open their eyes and look at you. But if you keep trying, and you keep centring yourself, and really look at that person, and really mirror their movements, maybe not this time but the next time you come you'll have a communication.'

TRUSTING TO THE MOMENT

One characteristic that both of these accounts have in common is that of capitalizing on the possibilities inherent in the moment. Neither I nor

Naomi Feil had any idea when we started how the attempts to communicate might develop. She had no guarantee that Gladys would begin to sing with her, and I could not have predicted that Bronwen would choose for the conversation to be a non-verbal one. Speaking for myself, I find a no-holds-barred, instant-response interaction both exciting and taxing. What I am also sure about, though, is that by setting aside all preconceptions one is entering fully into the world of the other person, and that means trusting to the moment to provide each way forward.

Elsewhere in the same video in which the interaction with Gladys occurs, Naomi Feil is shown interacting with another person, Mrs C, who has virtually no language left. It is a much shorter session, but Naomi Feil accompanies it with a commentary, which I have transcribed. This is not offered as a clearly structured piece of prose, but rather as a vivid account of process, with the ideals behind the work insightfully presented:

> When I did mention children her eyes brightened up, but then she left it, and what stimulated the togetherness I don't know, whether it was the children or not. I didn't know if it was the children, I didn't know if it was her mother. I know for a moment that she was with her mother, then she let that go. So we went from one thing to another, and I couldn't say what it was but there was a click, like now we're two human beings and we're together. I don't know what precipitated it really.
>
> Relating to her, to Mrs C, was difficult, first because I had a hard time getting eye-contact, and I didn't know what she was referring to, and I didn't know what was in her mind, but I knew there was something there, and that I needed to go wherever she was, and then we would have the basic communication that would connect, that the two of us would become one, even though it was a non-verbal communication. (TMK Productions and Memory Bridge 2007)

I should, perhaps, draw attention to the one way in which the Bronwen and Gladys sessions are contrasting. Whereas I entered into the dialogue with no desire to lead Bronwen in any direction, but rather to discover in which direction she wished to go, Naomi Feil on this occasion was determined, using all the strategies at her command, to awaken a response. We do not know how things might have turned out if I had decided on a technique familiar to me for drawing someone like Bronwen out. Nor do we know, if Naomi Feil had adopted an undirected approach, how Gladys might have responded. Both approaches are valid. I do know that it was essential to me to have no knowledge of Bronwen before meeting with her, as no doubt it was essential to Naomi Feil to have done her homework, or she would not have been able to tap into Gladys's religious belief. And it follows from this that Naomi Feil, using a proactive approach, would call upon such tools as talking and singing, whereas I was limited to the demands of Bronwen, who was in charge of the session.

SPIRITUALITY

The question arises as to what extent the two interactions described in detail above are exemplars of spirituality. With the communication of Naomi and Gladys the answer is an obvious one. If one defines spirituality in terms of orthodox religious belief, then this satisfies the criteria. But is there an element of the spiritual here over and above the overtly religious and, if so, in what terms are we to describe it? With the communication between myself and Bronwen there is no religious context available. So what, in spiritual terms, is going on here?

If one adopts the definition of spirituality proposed by Froggatt and Moffitt (1997, p.225) one may come a little closer to pinpointing the area we are exploring:

> Defining spirituality is always tricky. In this context we mean the search for that which gives zest, energy, meaning and identity to a person's life, in relation to other people, and to the wider world. Spirituality can be experienced in feelings of awe or wonder, those moments of life which take you beyond the mundane into a sacred place.

I would suggest that the interactions described earlier fulfil both of the conditions outlined here. Both myself and Naomi Feil embarked on separate adventures of discovery into the person and what was meaningful for them, and we would both assert that the intimacy we experienced was a profound interconnectedness with another human being, which enriched our lives and, though we cannot prove this, the lives of those with whom we interacted.

How common are these experiences? Probably rather rare. From observation of people with dementia in hospitals, nursing homes and in their own homes, I would suggest that most people with the condition are currently being denied the opportunity to interact in spiritual ways. Their lives seem to be confined to the mundane, and the practical level is not one on which they are likely to shine. What is needed is supporters (relatives, professional carers, volunteers) prepared to take the risk involved in deep communication and surrender to the moment. Ironically, time (the lack of) is often offered as the reason why interactions are not attempted, yet neither of those described took longer than seven minutes. Nothing less than a revolution in attitudes seems called for.

RELATIONSHIP

There follow some brief reports from various sources of successful forays into this territory. The first comes from a counsellor with many years' experience of working one-to-one with individuals with the diagnosis of dementia:

> Occasionally, and more often than I would have at first thought possible, our communication takes place within the myriad realms of silence. In those positive encounters I imagine it akin to a beautiful prism being held aloft between us; tantalizing in its elusive beauty, inviting wonder and interest. As a prism reflects multiple facets of light and colour, alighting here and there, so too can silence reflect multiple facets of personality, meaning and spirit, separateness and communion. (Lipinska 2009, p.100)

Lois McCloskey is an American musician who has worked extensively with people with dementia, and describes the approach as follows:

> I believe presence is the key element in working with people whose verbal skills are minimal. By presence I mean listening without a particular expectation or a prior agenda. Instead of trying to bring them to my world or orienting them to my 'reality', I allow myself to go where they are and orient myself to their reality. I look deep into their eyes and observe their facial expressions, their body postures, their behaviour. I speak quietly, calmly, and in a non-threatening tone. To do this I must be focused and free from distractions. (McCloskey 1990, p.63)

And here are three quotations from family carers. The message they share adds a further perspective to the idea of spiritual sharing: the benefits for those who make the effort of openness and adaptation.

> Mother was different, and discovering who she was each day was a delight. The bitterness she had lived with was draining from her mind…and in its place was a new pleasant outlook that seemed to surprise and please us both. More than once she gave me a loving look and simply whispered 'thank you'. These were the rewards I had missed in my childhood and were so welcome now. (Vogler 2003, p.37)

I sink into my mother's face like she is a meditation. We smile at each other for a half-hour, something we have never done before, something that would be too intense, too personal in our earlier, rational life together. Then her eyes gently flutter shut. I feel like I've been on a mystical retreat. I feel a rich sense of renewal and hope. (Shouse 2007, pp.125–126)

It's such a big mystery, living in suspended animation like this. But there is a kind of grace involved… When you do something for someone with Alzheimer's they forget it as soon as it's done, so you know you're not doing for credit. It's a kind of sacrament. (Peterson 2004, p.194)

LIVING IN THE MOMENT

All the above quotations refer to relationship, and that is where the greatest need is, and the greatest benefits are to be derived. But there is also the long-term enhancement of the carer's (family or professional) life from coming to terms with living in the moment. Anne Davis Basting enumerates some of these in the following passage:

Spending time with people who have dementia has made me a more patient parent, friend, daughter, sister, wife. It's made me notice and be endlessly thankful for things like the horizon of Lake Michigan, gray storm clouds, three or four well-chosen notes on a cello, and breathing. (Basting 2009, p.160)

I hope I have provided sufficient illustrations of the potential for close communication with individuals with dementia to convince the reader that this is not just an area worthy of exploration but a channel for spiritual insights that are difficult to access in any other way. My examples have mainly been individuals with more advanced dementia, because they are the most difficult to reach, and if I can show that there are real possibilities here, then my case for similar approaches to others at earlier stages of the condition is already made.

I want to refer back to the ideas presented at the outset from Zen Buddhism and the mindfulness branch of positive psychology. It seems supremely ironical that the ideals postulated by these contemporary movements should apparently find fulfilment in an aspect of the experience of people with dementia, and achieved without any effort or theorising on their part! This is certainly a phenomenon that demands further investigation.

Dementia has turned the concept of time on its head, and in the same film, *There is a Bridge* (TMK Productions and Memory Bridge 2007), which I have already drawn extensively upon, there is an interview with Stanley Hauerwas, a professor of theological ethics, in which he makes a passionate plea for deep communion: 'We forget that our most precious gift for one another is presence... To become a friend with someone with Alzheimer's is exactly the kind of challenge that it means to become a friend of time.'

NOTES

1. *When Your Heart Wants to Remember* (1999) was a film produced jointly by the BBC and the Royal College of Nursing. It was shown on BBC2 three times and then made commercially available. It is currently out of print.

2. *There is a Bridge* (2007) is available as a DVD produced by TMK Productions and Memory Bridge.

CHAPTER 6

To Live and Do and Help – A Life that's Worthwhile

Reflections on the Spiritual Meaning of Generosity for People Living with Dementia

Padmaprabha Dalby

INTRODUCTION

> 'I've really wanted to live…live and do and help, and have a life that's worthwhile, and then it all got taken away, absolutely all of it.'

These words describe one person's experience of a phase in her journey of living with dementia. She was a participant in a qualitative research study I conducted looking at the lived experience of spirituality and dementia. The participants were a small number of people with mild to moderate dementia who also had a significant spiritual or religious life. One of the striking outcomes was the participants' common emphasis upon generosity and helping others as part of their spiritual life, and the way in which having dementia had affected their capacity to give and help. The present chapter focuses on this aspect of the data and offers some reflections on the importance of generosity as an aspect of spirituality and as a means of supporting the personhood of people with dementia.

A BRIEF DESCRIPTION OF THE RESEARCH

The research reported here was undertaken as an in-depth study of the experience of spirituality and religion in people living with mild to moderate dementia. 'Spirituality' was defined as being concerned with creating and searching for meaning in life in the context of a person's relationship to the self and what is held sacred. 'Religion' was defined as the socially created context in which that search may be placed. Following Hill and

Pargament (2003), 'the sacred' was a broad and poetic term used to include people's experience of God, the Divine, 'ultimate reality' or that which transcends normal, everyday boundaries and experiences. As such, the understanding of spirituality adopted was a broad one, with the intention of including in the research anyone who felt themselves to have a spiritual and/or religious life that was personally significant.

My interest was in exploring with people who were living with dementia how their experience of spirituality or religion was affected by living with dementia, and how they felt living with dementia was affected by doing so in the context of a spiritual or religious life.

A qualitative research design was used and the interview transcripts were analysed using Interpretive Phenomenological Analysis (IPA). IPA is concerned with understanding the meaning of the research topic for individuals. There is the assumption that meaning is derived through the process of a social interaction between the participant and the researcher, in which both are engaged in a process of reflection on the subject (Smith 1997). The person's lived experience is not necessarily transparent within the data, but is sought through an analytical process on the part of the researcher (Smith, Jarman and Osborn 1999), who reads and re-reads the interview transcripts to identify significant themes for individuals and across the participant group. As the researchers in this method use themselves and their own knowledge and experience very fully, it is important that their personal and professional perspectives are acknowledged and held up to the light of reflection. I brought to this research my personal knowledge and experience of many years of Buddhist practice, as well as my passion as a clinical psychologist to hear the voices of people with dementia in their own right, rather than being spoken for by others.

The participants were recruited through Alzheimer's Society branches and through mental health clinicians within the National Health Service. Although information and requests for participants were also circulated widely to religious/spiritual groups and community centres, I found that people were reluctant to come forward without the reassurance of a personal/professional connection. This meant that all the participants were invited to take part in the research by my colleagues and professional acquaintances. When individuals did volunteer for the research, I followed a careful process of gaining informed consent and ensuring that a plan was in place if they should become distressed in the course of the interview, before commencing with the interview itself. All of the participants consented to publication of the outcomes of the research, including illustrative quotations, as long as the published material did not reveal their identities.

Six people were interviewed in the study. This is a small number so caution should be taken regarding generalising the findings. However, the results presented a rich picture of the experience of spirituality, religious faith and dementia for the people taking part.

THE PARTICIPANTS

Here follow brief pen pictures of the people who were interviewed, with key information (including names) changed or disguised to protect their identities. The age range was from early seventies to early nineties. All but 'Jeannie' were white British.

'Alma' had lived with Alzheimer's disease for about three years. She lived in her own home and was supported by family. She followed the teachings of an Indian guru and had a universal approach to faith and spirituality, believing that all paths led to the same spiritual experience or destination. She meditated daily and read spiritual literature. In her working life she had fulfilled a number of professional roles, mainly supporting or teaching children.

'Christine' had lived with Alzheimer's disease for about one year. She lived with her husband and had a large extended family. She had been a Christian through most of her life and this had given her strength in her professional life as a nurse. She attended a local church but had found it more difficult to take part in the life of the church community since the development of her memory problems.

'Breda' had lived with the effects of vascular dementia for about one year. She lived alone and had an independent and private lifestyle. She was a practitioner of spiritual healing, involving an active meditative practice that she had found difficult since the development of her symptoms. She had lost touch with many of her friends in the 'healing' world but had recently started to attend a local church. Professionally, she had been a teacher for many years.

'Peter' was living with early vascular dementia following a stroke some years earlier. He lived in a care home and was closely supported by his wife. He was a retired Christian minister, having converted to Christianity in his youth. He was still actively engaged in the life of the local church, as well as carrying out his own practice of personal and shared prayer for others.

'Jeannie' had a mixed diagnosis of vascular dementia and Alzheimer's disease and was living with distressing symptoms of delusions and paranoia in addition to the more common memory problems. She was a British Asian lady who had grown up overseas and been a Christian all her life. She attended church intermittently and prayed and read her Bible on her own. She had brought up a family and worked as a nurse.

'Gwen' had lived with Alzheimer's disease for about three years. She lived in a supported environment and was also supported by family. She had converted to Christianity as a young woman and lived much of her life overseas with her family, working as a nurse and missionary. She attended church and also prayed actively for others and read her Bible on her own.

As may be noticed, all of the participants had a history of working in 'helping professions'. As the participants were self-selecting, this was an interesting coincidence. It followed that giving to and helping others was of central importance to the participants. In fact, it became clear that these were aspects of their spirituality and of their identity as persons, as will be described in more detail below. It was also of note that the people interviewed had particularly strong religious or spiritual convictions.

A BRIEF OVERVIEW OF THE RESULTS

For the group as a whole, five superordinate themes were identified. These were 'experience of faith', 'searching for meaning in dementia', 'I'm not as I was – changes and losses in experience of the self', 'staying intact' and 'current pathways to spiritual connection and expression'. Each theme gathered together a number of subordinate themes. As these have been described in some depth elsewhere (Dalby, Sperlinger and Boddington forthcoming), the current chapter will focus on the aspects of these themes that featured giving and helping as part of a spiritual life.

GIVING AND HELPING AS AN ASPECT OF SPIRITUALITY

The majority of the group described their experience of faith as having continuity through their lives and as not being separate from life. Continuity was mainly experienced in the individuals' experience of and relationship with God or the Divine, which persisted regardless of having dementia; however, there was also continuity in the 'work' of spirituality. For example, Gwen said, 'My practical work is finished but my spiritual work is certainly not stopped,' and in making the point that spirituality was not separate from life, Breda said that spirituality was 'so much part of the work and how it's naturally used for the healing…I don't see it as separate'. For these women, the work of spirituality was tied up with helping others, either through practical means or through prayer.

All respondents communicated the spiritual values that they held dear and tried to live by. These included love, service, giving, being of use and sharing their faith with others. The quotations that follow, in which minor hesitations have mostly been removed, serve as illustrations:

- 'It's like a little motto I have – love all and serve all – and that gets you through a lot of things.' (Alma)

- 'Part of my reason for going into nursing was I thought there was something I could do in this world, you know, help other people and that sort of thing.' (Christine)

- 'I like doing something useful and especially, erm, the spiritual aspect.' (Breda)

- 'It was something really strong in me and that I felt I should share [my experience of Christianity], like I'm sharing to you.' (Gwen)

LOSSES AND SUPPORTS IN PERSONAL AND SPIRITUAL INTEGRITY

In carrying out the research, I was constantly struck by the losses and changes that most of the respondents experienced in their sense of themselves and their relationships with others. These gathered together in the theme 'I'm not as I was – changes and losses in experience of the self'. These losses seemed to be balanced by the efforts of the respondents, their families and friends to help the person 'stay intact'. In naming the theme 'staying intact', I acknowledged Joan Erikson's (1995, 1997) reflections upon the potential ninth stage of psychosocial development, in which an older person is faced with maintaining their wholeness and integrity in the face of the dissolutions of the physical body – and in the case of dementia, the gradual dissolution also of the experience of self. In a critical review of research into aspects of personhood in dementia, O'Connor *et al.* (2007) highlight the theme of profound loss running through descriptions of the subjective experience of dementia, as well as the issues of threats to, and preservation of, the self and sense of identity. The present research concurred with this.

In the current group, the themes of change, loss and staying intact were, in many cases (though not exclusively), tied up with giving to, caring for and helping others. Despite the losses, there was also a strong theme of gratitude for some. I would like to share here some examples from each person's story.

Alma

Alma felt a loss in her sense of independence and agency, her capacity to live, learn and explore as an individual. She described this as being 'like a parcel' – a rich metaphor of a person who is wrapped up, inhibited and unable to reveal and express her potential. I was fascinated, then, by her frequent remembrance of herself as a younger person. She told me many stories of her professional life and the value and enjoyment she found in helping others: 'I've been lucky – I've always had jobs I'd do for a hobby.' She was not the only person who reminisced with me, and I came to understand these stories as a way in which the respondents recollected themselves and, what was most important to them, a strategy to help them stay intact. Alma still managed to live out her wish to help others. She told me, 'I've got a couple of charities' – a phrase that seemed to express the importance of charitable giving for her sense of herself as a person. She had chosen charities that helped support the learning of young and troubled people, just as she had done practically in her earlier life.

Interviewing Alma was a poignant experience as there was the touching sadness of her sense of loss, yet she was also a joyful person who continued to embrace and love life even as she looked forward with clear eyes to her own death. She was one of the people who expressed a sense of gratitude or being blessed: 'I've had so many blessings you see. I've got a nice home and lovely family and you can't help getting old. So it's lucky if you're born with some gifts that get you through life.'

Christine

Christine had been led by her faith to become a nurse as a way to help others. Now she felt acutely the loss of her capacity to help others in practical ways, as a result of being less reliable and less able to remember what was asked of her:

> 'when I say I will do something for someone and I will forget, and I hate being unreliable because I've never been. If someone gives me something to do, and then I can't remember whether I've done it or not, then I really get…yes, end up getting in quite a silly state about it.'

Christine was trying to cope with this through a range of both practical and emotional strategies, including trying to cover up her lapses. She had also withdrawn from situations in which her difficulties might be exposed, such as groups at her church, and was becoming somewhat socially isolated as a result:

'I hope it will never become so isolating that I don't socialise at all, but I am aware that it is one of those things about Alzheimer's that you do become socially, I don't mean to sound dramatic, outcast.'

Breda

Breda had experienced a dramatic loss in her ability to carry out spiritual healing. As she had found the onset of her cognitive problems such a shock and so debilitating, she described herself as being 'a mess':

'Since, I've been a mess, I haven't been able to do it, because what you have to do is hold the link between yourself and the Divine and the person you're working on...so I pulled out...I really withdrew from life.'

As a result of her withdrawal, Breda had entered a process of deep personal questioning concerning what she could learn from her experience. She had concluded that she had developed her symptoms as part of her spiritual 'life plan', as an opportunity to develop compassion for others with difficulties. She reflected on how she had the practical skills to help people but had lacked the corresponding compassion, and she believed that she would be able to continue on her path once she had learned this lesson.

Breda had chosen to take part in the research because she had seen the opportunity to help. She experienced this, in itself, as a spiritual gift to her. So, as well as giving to others through her participation, she expressed gratitude for the opportunity to do so. She spoke of how I had 'served her well' by listening to her and allowing her to give to others through her experience.

'I thought "Oh! Maybe at last I'll be of some use because I am experienced in this mess!" And I could, if I was given the strength... that I've got the focus to enable the answers to come for you, I was going to say for your purpose, it's not very well worded but that we'd be able to communicate. You see, I haven't been lucid like this for I can't tell you how long!'

Peter

Peter was the one person who did not communicate a sense of loss in relation to himself or his situation. He had an attitude of taking 'one week at a time' and had perhaps reached a sense of acceptance in relation to his health that protected him from feelings of loss. Like Alma, Peter recollected his life of giving to others and spoke with some emotion of the part he played in taking Christianity to other countries. He also communicated that it was important to him to be remembered by others for the work that he did.

Peter actively participated in his church community and communicated the importance of praying for others and being prayed for. He had a prayer list and prayed for people in it twice a day – once alone and once in a shared practice with his wife.

Jeannie

For Jeannie, much of the sense of loss was focused on her changed relations with others, some of which had become more conflictual. However she also spoke of her reduced ability to share her faith in the way that she once did, due to memory problems and trouble expressing herself:

> 'I never press or push anybody to believe, they've all got their faiths...
> but if they ask me what's my belief, I tell them. Even I'm getting bad at
> it now as I don't remember as I used to, so if I forget I say "I'm so sorry,
> I can't remember."'

One of the striking elements of Jeannie's interview was her extensive expression of gratitude. She spoke of gratitude to God as being the main thing that sustained her through her difficulties. She also spoke of the benefits of receiving help from someone who is 'open and clean in their heart'. Reflecting upon Jeannie's perspective made me think about the openness of heart that arises in both gratitude and giving, and the human connection that follows.

Gwen

Gwen had given her life to others and the service of God, as this is what she had felt she was being told to do in her early conversion experience: 'I [thought] "Is that what I ought be doing?" And the longer I prayed the stronger it got and I could not turn round and not do it.'

She did not experience a loss in relation to her missionary work, as she felt that she continued to do what God asked of her and she also looked back on the life she had lived with gladness at having served, as she saw it, God's purpose for her.

> 'I know I can't go back anymore. I can't go roaming around the country
> anymore...but I can still pray for everything, every person. I'm praying

for people that I've no idea who they are but I'm praying for them, that they will go ahead with…what God wants them to be. But looking back at it, I'm glad…I'm glad that I did what I did. A big help. A big help now. When I get up now sometimes, I can't remember what the day is, silly things like that, but I think "Well Lord, you know what you're doing."'

REFLECTIONS: OTHER RESEARCH FINDINGS

This is not the only research to identify that people with dementia want to continue helping others. In studies that explored the subjective experience of dementia, Menne, Kinney and Morhardt (2002) and Beard (2004) found that helping others or being of use to others was a key strategy in helping people to retain continuity in their lives and support their sense of self. In a study of the social meaning of living with dementia (Langdon, Eagle and Warner 2007), participants spoke of their lack of use to society, which had a negative effect on their self-esteem. The authors found participants keen to help others by taking part in the study.

Giving and personhood

Kitwood (1997a) defined personhood as 'a standing or status that is bestowed on one human being, by others, in the context of relationship and social being. It implies recognition, respect and trust' (p.8).

From the examples discussed in this chapter, it is easy to see how the participants' changed perceptions of their own capacity to help affected their sense of themselves in the social world and therefore, potentially, their sense of personhood.

Love, generosity and altruism are core values at the heart of many of the world's religions. So it should hardly be surprising that people who have lived out spiritual or religious values for much of their lives should wish to continue to give to others, and experience grief and loss when this proves difficult. The difficulties may be due to the changing cognitive capacities of the person (for example Christine, who could not remember what her friends had asked her to do), but they may also have a social element. Does society, and do spiritual communities, see people living with dementia as still having something of value to give? Once giving and helping become difficult, the consequences touch a number of aspects of human experience: there is loss of the personal satisfaction and sense of achievement involved in giving, loss of the human connection that is created, loss of the social standing and status conferred and loss of, or challenge to, the spiritual benefits.

The spiritual meaning of giving

The spiritual meaning of giving may vary somewhat according to differing religious or spiritual beliefs. Speaking from my own spiritual perspective, in Buddhist teachings a generous heart is said to be a great treasure. Spiritual emotions such as generosity and gratitude flow from a deep understanding that material wealth or worldly status cannot be held onto and that spiritual wealth comes from the peace of living in harmony with the flux and flow of ultimate reality. Through the acts of both giving (giving materially, giving energy or time, or giving spiritually through prayer, meditation or teachings) and receiving with an open heart, individuals acknowledge, and become more aware of, the interconnectedness of humanity. Experiencing, and living in harmony with, this interconnectedness, we become less inclined to hold tight to a fixed concept of 'me' and 'mine', which Buddhism teaches us is the delusion of a small mind. I imagine that, although doctrines may vary from one religious perspective to another, the central themes of letting go of worldly wealth and experiencing human interconnectedness are universal. When an individual's very sense of self is threatened by the experience of dementia, one can imagine the human and spiritual benefits of generosity and gratitude.

CONCLUSIONS

I believe this research and the reflections promoted by it offer a particular challenge to spiritual communities. How do we promote attitudes and opportunities to enable people with dementia to continue to give and connect, as valued members of spiritual communities? The respondents here have given a snapshot of some of the ways that the values of generosity and love can continue to find expression: personal communication, charitable giving, prayer, remembrance of achievements and relationships, and continued development and transformation of spiritual emotions (for example, Breda developing compassion and Alma and Jeannie staying in touch with gratitude). They have also given us a glimpse of the social isolation that may follow when a person's spiritual aspirations to give and help are thwarted.

Concluding this chapter, I find myself reflecting again on Breda's remark which I quoted at the beginning: 'I've really wanted to live...a life that's worthwhile.' Most, if not all, spiritual and religious perspectives recognise the unique value and worth of every individual. How do we help everyone contribute and connect to enrich our world? I personally was enriched by engaging in the conversations and analysis that were at the heart of this research. I hope that this chapter, in turn, will enrich others and inspire them to help people with dementia live a life that's worthwhile.

ACKNOWLEDGMENTS

The research reported in this chapter was conducted in partial fulfilment of the requirements of Canterbury Christ Church University for the degree of Doctor of Clinical Psychology and was undertaken whilst I was in the employ of Sussex Partnership NHS Foundation Trust. Thanks are due to Dr David Sperlinger and Steve Boddington, who supervised and supported me, and to Dr Fiona Pipon-Young, who carried out a credibility check on the data. Thanks are also due to the six participants who generously shared their experience.

CHAPTER 7

Voicing the Spiritual

Working with People with Dementia

Harriet Mowat

INTRODUCTION

As I write this chapter in June 2010, I am sitting in my 81-year-old father-in-law's house, waiting for him to prepare to visit his wife of 55 years who is having a hip replacement in the local hospital. The reason I am here is not because he is unable to manage himself. Despite chronic heart disease and diabetes he has the capacity to cook, clean and care for himself. He is able to read and write and socialise. His unspoken reason for wanting me with him was to accompany him with his fears and anxieties. The way he described this was to say that he was not looking forward to being alone while Mum was in hospital. These anxieties are related to his age and Mum's age. His unarticulated fear that Mum would not survive the operation; that he would collapse during the night (which he has done before) and no one would be there to help him; that he might find himself alone and lonely; that he might find himself pondering the meaning of his life and need reassurance that his life had been worth it. It was these fears that prompted him to change his mind about refusing previous offers of help and declare that he would like someone with him. His needs are spiritual. He needs to know that he is loved and that he can rely on someone else to help him if necessary. He needs someone to attend to his fears in a way that does not make them worse. He needs a listener and he needs a space to express his fears. That is why I'm sitting at his dining room table waiting for him to get ready to visit the hospital.

This chapter is about creating the conditions for *expressive space* so that a spiritual conversation can take place if required. It reports a particular project which focused on doing so with people who, unlike my father-in-law, have cognitive challenges in the form of some kind of dementia.

AGEING IS A SPIRITUAL MATTER: WE ARE ALL INVOLVED

Mark Buchanan (2002) writes that having a sense of other and a sense of missing something is part of our human condition. Ageing is an opportunity for us to ponder this 'miss'. We all have spiritual needs at any age. These needs include finding meaning or purpose in our lives, having hope, being loved and being able to love, being accepted for what we are, being forgiven and forgiving, feeling valued and being able to transcend our daily lives (Lachlan 2010). As we age, our 'groanings' (Job 3:24; Romans 8:26) become more pressing and less easy to avoid. We consider our legacy and our succession. Life becomes shorter and meanings become more elusive. People with dementia are no different in this respect.

It is important to note at the outset that we are *all* ageing and *all* spiritual beings. Spirituality is present in all human beings. Those writers interested in children's spirituality, such as Brendan Hyde (2008), David Hay and Rebecca Nye (2006) and Kate Adams, Brendan Hyde and Richard Woolley (2008) show in their research how children demonstrate an innate spiritual sensitivity, which Hay (2006) in particular suggests is socialised out of us as we grow into adolescence. Jung (Jung and Read 1960) argues that we must then spend the second half of our life trying to retrieve that sensitivity. Betty Friedan (1993) notes in her seminal work on the advantages of ageing that:

> Only a few very wise psychological theorists in their own old age have said flatly like Jung, that problems are likely if we try to live the afternoon of life by the chart of the morning…Jung felt that the older person must devote serious attention to the inner life. Jung insisted that aging individuals run into difficulties when they refuse to see that the second half of life is not governed by the same principles as the first. (Friedan 1993, p.122)

Friedan was prompted to write her book on age after noting that both she and her contemporaries were reluctant to recognise ageing as something happening to them, or to see it in any way as to be welcomed. The discipline of gerontology itself distanced personal ageing from ageing that happened to others. This arguably held up the acceptance of ageing for a generation and influenced the emphasis on the 'problem' of ageing.

The hard facts are that we are *all* ageing and we are *all* vulnerable to cognitive impairment. Carers, cared for, professional health and social care staff are all involved in the same human processes.

SPIRITUAL TALK IS OCCASIONAL, UNEXPECTED AND POWERFUL

Like my father-in-law, most people do not generally embark on discussions about the meaning in and of their lives. We do not generally talk about the spiritual as a discrete and identifiable process. Instead, spiritual matters, insights and anxieties 'pop up' as a consequence of other discussion. The spiritual attender needs to be mindful of the sporadic, fragmented nature of spiritual discussion; its apparently *ad hoc* and surprising appearance and the serendipitous nature of that appearance. It is important to allow space for spiritual discussion and to recognise it when it appears.

SPIRITUAL CARE AND SPIRITUAL NEED

The aim of the project in which I have been involved was to work with older people with dementia and their carers to develop, put into practice and review a spiritual care 'intervention'. It was aimed at helping older people with dementia and their carers to remain connected with their communities and their spiritual lives, and at supporting staff working with older people in recognising older people's spiritual needs. The project was funded in 2008 by the Mental Wellbeing in Later Life unit of the Scottish Government.

The definition of spiritual care and needs spelled out in the Scottish Executive (2002b) *Health Directive Letter* was used. This states that:

> Spiritual care is usually given in a one to one relationship, is completely person-centred and makes no assumptions about personal conviction or life orientation. Religious care is given in the context of the shared religious beliefs, values and liturgies and lifestyle of a faith community. Spiritual care is not necessarily religious. Religious care at its best should always be spiritual.

SPIRITUAL CARE IS PART OF HOLISTIC CARE

This project started from the recognition of a growing body of knowledge that shows that spiritual practices are linked to positive wellbeing and mental health (Koenig, McCullough and Larson 2001; Lachlan 2007; Larson, Sawyers and McCullough 1997; Mowat 2007; Pargament 2002).

The report *With Health in Mind* (Scottish Executive 2002a) emphasises the importance of being able to reflect on and understand life events, which is enhanced by the 'personal capacity and resilience that a spiritual life frequently provides'. This is echoed in the Scottish Executive's further report, *Equal Minds*, which addresses the mental health inequalities in Scotland (Myers, McCollam and Woodhouse 2005, p.18). It states that 'mental health is the emotional and spiritual resilience which allows us to enjoy life and to survive pain, disappointment and sadness' and cites as one of the protective factors for individuals 'being spiritual with access to faith groups'.

The Mental Health and Wellbeing in Later Life report (NHS Health Scotland, 2004) notes the effect that social isolation has on individuals and stresses the importance of self-help and peer support. It has been shown that a focus on spiritual needs can make a significant contribution to personal wellbeing alongside the support it lends to community connectedness. The report draws on the widespread consultation undertaken, which listed faith and/or spiritual practices amongst the coping strategies identified by individuals and the value placed on person-centred care.

This evidence substantiates the Scottish Government's recognition that spirituality is of importance in the lives of individuals within the health service and wider communities. Spiritual care is now a positive requirement within the Health Service (Scottish Executive 2002b), but there needs to be a much stronger emphasis on this dimension within community-based activity.

The project described below is relevant to the current policy initiatives expressed in the document *All our Futures* (Scottish Government 2007) where commitments are made to a vision of a Scotland where ageing is welcomed and adaptation and positive approaches to ageing are encouraged. Recently the Shifting the Balance of Care initiative (NHS Health Scotland 2005) has highlighted the importance of re-thinking the relationship between hospital and community.

USING PRACTICAL THEOLOGICAL REFLECTION TO ENCOURAGE SPIRITUAL CARE

There were three people in our spiritual care team: Jim Simpson, a healthcare chaplain; Fran Marquis, an artist; and Harriet Mowat (myself), a qualitative writer. We met regularly and the writer asked the two practitioners to keep a diary of their interactions and the events. The qualitative writer utilised the reflective cycle to stimulate thinking and progress action.

We used a practical theological research framework developed by Swinton and Mowat (2006) which incorporates an action research cycle and theological reflection. This framework incorporates critical reflection on spiritual practices and data collection using social science qualitative methods, and is intended to generate revised forms of spiritual practice as a consequence of careful data collection, analysis and reflection. This involved finding out what the current situation was, encouraging full participation by the groups of older people and their carers and the staff, and allowing participants rather than the spiritual careworkers to dictate the speed and content of the interventions. The framework is illustrated in Figure 7.1.

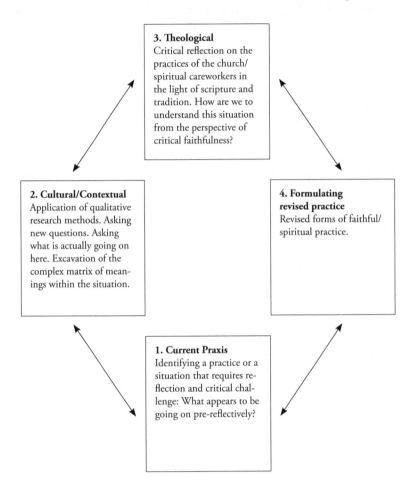

3. Theological
Critical reflection on the practices of the church/ spiritual careworkers in the light of scripture and tradition. How are we to understand this situation from the perspective of critical faithfulness?

2. Cultural/Contextual
Application of qualitative research methods. Asking new questions. Asking what is actually going on here. Excavation of the complex matrix of meanings within the situation.

4. Formulating revised practice
Revised forms of faithful/ spiritual practice.

1. Current Praxis
Identifying a practice or a situation that requires reflection and critical challenge: What appears to be going on pre-reflectively?

Figure 7.1 Theological reflection model

We worked across one region in Scotland with drop-in groups, lunch clubs, residential homes and day care settings. These were run by a variety of voluntary groups. The spiritual care team were 'reactive' rather than proactive in approach. They responded to the mood of the group and fitted in with that, rather than arriving with any preconceptions or rigid plan.

The spiritual careworkers spent time visiting and discussing with the various groups, all of whom were providing community-based services for older people with dementia. They collected notes after each encounter. These notes were written up as part of the reflective process and the narrative of the project. The spiritual care team 'embedded' themselves in these groups and helped develop activities which emerged organically from the participants. This process took time and required constant review of needs and wishes.

CREATING EXPRESSIVE SPACE FOR THE SPIRITUAL

We developed a process and framework for 'accessing and working with the spiritual' with people with dementia, their carers, volunteers and paid staff. This framework emerged out of the development work that we carried out. It is informed by wider reading and discussion and is an expression of good practice in spiritual care. The framework involves entering into and building relationships so that a spiritual 'conversation' can be maintained.

The framework (Figure 7.2) is described diagrammatically and explained thereafter.

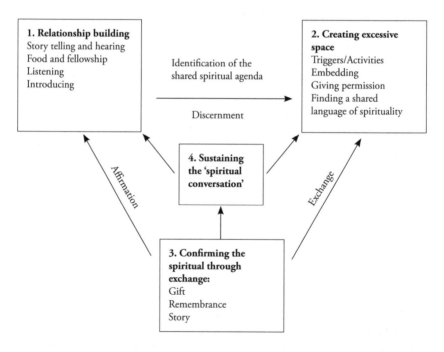

Figure 7.2 Accessing the spiritual framework

This framework is based on the assumption that spiritual matters are mediated through relationships with others and with God. God is understood very differently by us all. Whatever our concept of God, however, we develop it through our relationships with our fellow human beings.

BUILDING THE RELATIONSHIP

The first task of accessing the spiritual is to build relationships. In the case of our project we did this both in groups and with individuals. The spiritual careworkers spent time and energy in 'getting to know' the individuals in the groups. The importance of being able to name individuals in the group and to remember their names is a spiritual task in itself. Naming gives identity and recognition.

The way we identified ourselves was relevant to the way in which a spiritual conversation could develop. 'Jim the healthcare chaplain' gave permission for discussion about spiritual matters, and gave permission to declare no interest. Both were equally apparent. 'Fran the artist' allowed people to talk about their own artistic interests. 'Harriet the writer' encouraged people to tell stories.

The relationship-building involved hearing the stories of the groups and individuals and working with those stories. This often involved accounts of diagnosis and reaction to it, stories of decline and preparation for residential care, and stories of loss.

The spiritual relationship and the spiritual 'interventions' started as soon as we introduced ourselves and arrived in the group settings. We saw that the whole process, from the initial approach, was not so much a discrete intervention as a messy process. The activities that we thought would be interventions were in fact only markers along the way. The relationships that we built were part of a spiritual journey that we embarked upon together with the participating individuals, older people, paid staff and family carers. The building of the relationships *were* the interventions.

We discovered that the storytelling came out of good company, and in particular good food. Some of the groups specialised in good food and, depending on the seating arrangements, stories were batted back and forth.

Extract from diary notes

> 'W' is in day care and told me he cannot attend church any more. It is too difficult to concentrate but in the past he attended a Scottish Episcopal Church and was involved in the Scouting Troop. His eyes lit up when

he spoke of his friends and the activities that many years on were still meaningful for him.

'E' is in respite care and wanted to speak of her feelings of guilt. She has a loving family and many friends but when the 'darkness comes' and she feels depressed, begins to feel sorry for herself. How can she talk to her family about this? My visit provided the perfect opportunity to tell her story that has been locked somewhere deep inside for too long. We sat quietly when she said, 'thank you for listening!'

'A' is a keen singer who put everything she had into 'Climb every mountain' from *The Sound of Music*. I asked her why this song was special and she told of a visit (she couldn't remember where) to the country and seeing the sights. She spoke of the beauty and majesty and how this made her feel special. When she sang the song it was like reliving that wonder experience.

'K' is a carer whose partner lives with dementia. He is actively involved in making a support group work and at the same time dealing with his own emotional turmoil. At coffee time I listened to his story, including his fears for the future. In the space between busyness we met each other and he seemed to draw strength from me as he let down his guard, even if just for a few moments.

This first stage of the framework allowed us to start to discern the spiritual positions and understandings and backgrounds of the groups and individuals. Discernment is a key process in spiritual relationship-building. This helped us think through the most appropriate ways forward in terms of triggers and activities as part of the second step of the framework.

Extract from healthcare chaplain's notes

Watching people eat, sing and laugh together, I observed a kind of spirituality similar to any church gathering. Initially this surprised me, since I had not expected it, and if I had been dropped in from outer space and did not know this was an independent charity supported by social work, I would have thought it was a church/faith community. God was acknowledged in a grace, through my association with chaplaincy then later in Christmas carols. The people I have come to know appear loved and secure in each other's company. Carers are able to relax and trust their loved ones to one another, so sharing the responsibility for a time. More than one reference was made to 'H' who facilitates various groups and seems available 24/7 for advice and support. Even when one carer was away visiting a frail relative, 'H' kept in touch by phone. Such actions are appreciated and have a positive effect on the volunteers who share her vision.

There is undoubtedly a sense of belonging and perhaps people have found a new identity through their dementia. I was moved at the open display of emotion and how this was normal and acceptable. Through traditional music, a common heritage is explored, and in sharing gifts the bonds of friendship are strengthened. At times I felt like an outsider, but those around me would have been shocked if I had admitted it, they went out of their way to be inclusive and very generous with their welcome. At other times I felt really involved with those I knew, held hands and shared little stories of the day and expectations to come. It was a rich experience to be alongside such caring and cared for people.

This made me reflect on the spiritual intervention and I wonder if the chaplaincy role is to recognise where 'spirituality' already exists and through listening and questions to articulate people's hopes and fears. In a person-centred way it's about meeting people as a trained professional, comfortable with spiritual things and through a personality honed by experience of life issues. My role as a hospital chaplain seemed to make a difference.

CREATING EXPRESSIVE SPACE

This part of the framework focused on developing the opportunity for expressive space. The way this worked best was to provide some kind of activity – art work, singing, storytelling – that was intended to allow spiritual talk to flow. The spiritual careworkers tried out a variety of triggers and events. These are discussed in the next section. These events were managed in various ways and were a consequence of discussion and fitting in with the general group 'way'.

The expressive space made it possible for the spiritual to emerge. The skill of the spiritual careworkers meant that they could hear the spiritual. They were able to distinguish noise from signal. Examples of creating expressive space included singing, painting together, storytelling and eating together.

WEAVING TO CREATE EXPRESSIVE SPACE

This activity took a long while to develop and this gave it its strength. Over a period of weeks the spiritual careworkers visited the lunch club and engaged in general storytelling and listening. Once a relationship had developed that allowed trust and laughter to be its central features, it was suggested that Jim and Fran find a particular space in the busy lunch club routines to focus on spiritual matters. This could not have developed earlier in the process. The relationship-building allowed it to happen naturally.

On the day of the weaving we enjoyed a two-hour lunch of delicious soup and homemade bread. A striking feature of this group is that the carers and helpers have adopted the pace of the slowest. This required some slowing down on the part of the spiritual careworkers, and we noted how peaceful it was to take two hours over lunch. The lunch was served onto a large table around which we all sat, and there was much talk and fellowship demonstrated. Once lunch was cleared away there was a general re-arranging and visits to the facilities, and people then sat in a horseshoe looking at Jim, who was leading the session. The session started with Jim pointing out the importance of light, no matter how small, and lighting floating candles. He introduced the idea of the weaver and how our lives are all woven together, and after a couple of songs he invited people to choose a piece of cloth that attracted them from a basket of cloth strips he had collected earlier.

People then wove their piece of cloth into the frame and were encouraged to speak about the significance of the cloth to them. This took quite a while and there were several re-visits to choose a second piece of cloth or to re-weave the original. Everybody joined in and by the end there was quite a congestion, with people wanting to thread their cloth.

Jim and Fran then went around the group, showing the frame to each person and eliciting more comments and stories. We then sang another song and finished with a poem read by Jim.

After the formal finish of the session there was much more talk about the cloth strips and their meaning. One older woman went up to the frame on her way past to the tea trolley, touched her piece of cloth and said, 'That's my mother'.

CONFIRMING THE SPIRITUAL THROUGH EXCHANGE AND GIFT

The third stage in the framework is to develop the relationship so that it is 'normalised' and cherished through gift and exchange. For example, we returned paintings nicely framed to those who had done art work, we took photos of the individuals while they were working on their pieces and gave the participants their photos both of the groups and the individuals, and we returned to share meals and conversation and to continue the spiritual conversations by acts of remembrance. By this we mean that we made real efforts to remember and notice the occasional spiritual reference and keep this on the agenda. This attentive listening is also a spiritual care skill.

SUSTAINING THE CONVERSATION

The three stages described above revolve around and interact with the need to sustain and make explicit the spiritual nature of our selves. In order to be effective we need to be able to maintain the conversation over a period of time. This is something that staff and carers can pick up on. A project such as this one initiates changes that can be sustained by others with support.

Storytelling and listening dominated all the activities. The activities were a vehicle for the story. They were characterised by slow pace, review and revisiting, and by pleasure and laughter. The stories, of course, continue.

CHECKLIST FOR SUSTAINING SPIRITUAL CONVERSATIONS

As a result of these activities and events we drew up a checklist based on the framework that encourages groups to sustain spiritual conversations as part of their daily practice. It is intended as a way to prompt individuals and groups to focus on the spiritual aspects of their relationships.

- Are you making time to have conversations?

- Do you know everybody's name?

- Do you know something about all the people you work with in terms of their life experiences or background?

- Are you telling people about your own experiences?

- Can you remember something about a previous conversation with this group/this person?

- Have you eaten a meal, or shared food or drink with this group/ this person recently?

- Have you exchanged photos or tokens with this person or group?

- Is there prayer or shared contemplation in your relationship with this person or this group?

- What is the easiest context in which to connect with this person or group? (e.g. singing, dancing, garden, drinking coffee, etc.)

- How are you helping this person/this group with their spiritual lives?

SUMMARY

This project has highlighted the value of giving space and time for spiritual conversations. This value was felt alike by staff, carers, families and the people with dementia. It allows everybody to feel part of something and equally involved. It challenges the idea that older people with dementia are somehow 'other' than ourselves.

We noted that discussion about diagnosis was prevalent. People felt that the way they were told their diagnoses affected their future response and actions. With this in mind we conducted a further project using the expressive space framework and liaising with an interactive theatre group through Alzheimer's Scotland. This allowed some of the anxieties and difficulties around diagnosis telling and giving to be discussed and aired in a dramatic form. We asked old age psychiatrists who are involved in diagnosis telling to tell us their own stories of delivering news of dementia, so that their own perceptions and anxieties could be incorporated into the theatrical representation.

The framework developed could be used by other groups and is best seen as a general way in which spiritual conversation can be generated and supported.

Given the great importance to general wellbeing of investigating our inner lives and finding meaning, hope and love in the face of ill health and difficulties, this kind of approach to caring is a way of being for all concerned, one that fulfils our potentials as connected, loving people in relationship with others working to understand our meaning in the world.

CHAPTER 8

New Directions in Cognitive Behavioural Therapy for Older People with Dementia and Depression

Paul Green

RESTRICTED ACCESS TO SERVICES

Before considering the ways in which cognitive behavioural therapy (CBT) may be used to treat depression in clients with dementia, it is worth making some general points about older people's access to psychological therapies in the UK and the adaptations which might be required to meet their particular needs. It has been estimated that 25 per cent of older people living in the community experience symptoms of depression, a third discuss it with their GP and half of those receive treatment, which usually comprises medication (Department of Health 2008). Hilton (2009) estimates that 40 per cent of older people attending their GP surgery in any two-week period will be experiencing mental health problems. However, older people with emotional disorders are less likely to be offered psychological therapies than their younger counterparts, despite evidence which suggests that they may be more willing to discuss their difficulties than accept medication (Chew-Graham, Baldwin and Burns 2004). Time constraints may lead to under-recognition of this or, alternatively, a lack of awareness regarding the utility of psychological therapies for this client group may prevent older people from being referred when it is appropriate to do so.

Some therapists have suggested that older adults may not benefit from CBT because their 'fluid intelligence' or reasoning ability declines with age. However, Doubleday, King and Papageorgieu (2002) found that older adults with anxiety disorders who were randomly allocated to CBT showed no positive correlation between the significant reductions noted in their scores on the Beck Anxiety Inventory (Beck, Epstein, Brown and Steer 1988) and high levels of fluid intelligence.

CBT is a structured, problem-orientated psychological treatment in which clients are helped to understand maladaptive thoughts and behaviours and develop strategies to change them. A collaborative approach ensures that the client is an active participant in this process rather than a passive recipient of care. An important aspect of this is the selection of goals, which should be specific, achievable and measurable. This allows both therapist and client to match them to techniques, evaluate the impact of interventions and identify progress towards them (McGinn and Sanderson 2001). It appears that the highly focused and structured nature of CBT with its clear agenda allows clients to draw concrete and specific conclusions about their symptoms, even if their fluid intelligence has declined. It is therefore not too abstract or exploratory for people whose fluid intelligence may have declined.

Unfortunately, therapeutic pessimism often inhibits older people's access to psychological treatments (Hepple 2004), and mental health problems like depression are sometimes mistakenly regarded as a normal consequence of ageing. This was reflected in a joint report by the Healthcare Commission, Audit Commission and Commission for Social Care Inspection, which found that local and public services harboured deep-rooted cultural attitudes to ageing and its impact on mental health (Staffordshire University et al. 2008).

The design and development of the Improving Access to Psychological Therapies (IAPT) programme appears to focus on working-age adults with older people designated as a 'special interest area'. The outcome measures used have not been standardised or validated for use with the older adult population and the training provided has tended not to include any particular attention to their needs (Hilton 2009).

THE POTENTIAL VALUE OF CBT

However, specialist primary care psychological therapy services for older people are being developed in some areas, and it is hoped that this trend will continue. The evidence to date suggests that members of this client group are just as able to benefit from CBT as their younger counterparts. Laidlaw (2001) conducted an empirical review of the then literature and concluded that CBT produced the largest effect sizes of treatments within each study for late life depression. A more recent meta-analysis of 57 controlled intervention studies by Pinquart, Duberstein and Lyness (2007) found that CBT had stronger effects than Interpersonal Psychotherapy (IPT) and miscellaneous other interventions in the treatment of depressed older adults. The literature regarding CBT for older people with mental health problems is not extensive but indicates that 'The particular difficulties caused by adaptation to loss, bereavement and physical illness, depression, anxiety, cognitive impairment and carer stress may all respond to treatment using this approach' (Green 2006, pp.4–5).

There are various ways in which CBT can be adapted to suit the particular needs of older people and improve therapeutic outcomes. With regard to depression, for example, traditional models focus on negative aspects of self-appraisal and may fail to consider the role of positive beliefs which have previously served to maintain self-esteem. As they get older, most people change roles and goals without becoming depressed because they have functional self-beliefs which nourish a sense of worth. Depression may occur when there is a failure to reinforce these, combined with the development of negative self-beliefs. Assessing the client's dysfunctional negative ideas and pre-morbid functional belief system will help determine how a sense of worth was previously maintained and identify positive cognitions and coping strategies (James, Kendell and Reichelt 1999).

Some clients may associate old age exclusively with loss and degeneration, assuming that unhappiness is a normal part of ageing. CBT can be used to explore the socio-cultural context of growing older and challenge the negative assumptions they have internalised. It is important to take account of 'cohort beliefs', which may be defined as:

> the set of cultural norms, historical events and personal events that occurred during a specific generation… Understanding older people in terms of their generational cohort allows therapists a way of gaining insight into the societal norms and rules that may influence an individual's behaviour. The therapist may need to take account of the different cultural expectations regarding health-seeking behaviour among older adults as compared to younger adults, especially with regard to views on the care and treatment of conditions such as depression and anxiety. (Laidlaw *et al.* 2003, p.7)

The loss of highly valued roles and goals as a result of advancing age may make a person vulnerable to depression, and this should also be considered. However, older adults are the least homogeneous of all age groups, with more differences than similarities evident. Adaptations may be unnecessary, particularly among the younger of the two generations which make up the older adult population.

Cohort beliefs may include religious values which are more commonly held by older people. It is important for therapists to be able to work within the client's own frame of reference without the therapist's beliefs being involved in the process. CBT differs in this sense from therapies which operate from a particular spiritual stance, such as pastoral or Christian counselling. The client can be encouraged to draw upon a faith perspective if this is a source of strength or hope, but also supported to challenge beliefs which trigger feelings of guilt and self-blame. Dementia may pose a challenge to the sufferer's spiritual values and the neutral stance of the therapist can facilitate a non-judgemental exploration of this. People's beliefs may change as a result of the process but this is entirely the choice of the client. It is also important to remember that therapeutic modalities are not neutral and value-free in themselves but rooted in different ideologies, such as the empiricism which underpins CBT, and these should not be imposed on the client either.

CBT can also be adapted to facilitate adjustment to physical health problems which may occur in old age. The three dimensions of impairment, disability and handicap can be used to conceptualise the physical effects of illness, its effect on the person's ability to perform 'normal' activities and its social impact. 'In this tripartite framework, it is apparent that the way a person copes with the disability and handicap components is under much more conscious control by the individual as compared to the impairment component' (Laidlaw, Thompson and Gallagher-Thompson 2004, p.396). This is a concept which could usefully be applied to clients with a diagnosis of dementia, 40–50 per cent of whom experience depressive symptoms, with 17 per cent meeting the criteria for major depression (Lavretsky 2003). The experience of memory problems may trigger feelings of shame and embarrassment which result in a desire to prevent deficits from becoming apparent to others, leading to abandonment of activities and avoidance of social contact. This issue will be returned to in more detail later, but for the moment it is worth noting that the true extent of an individual's current level of impairment may be over-estimated by that person and exacerbated by symptoms of depression.

Teri and Gallagher-Thompson (1991) found that the absence of pleasurable experiences and the presence of aversive ones can trigger and maintain depression in people with dementia when they are no longer able to participate in previously valued activities and lose independence. They developed two CBT programmes, one with a cognitive focus for mildly impaired clients, and one with a behavioural focus, to be used with those more severely impaired and their carers. Teri et al. (1997) found that active behavioural treatments focused either on pleasant events (for clients with dementia) or on caregiver problem-solving produced a significant reduction in depressive symptoms for both parties of client/carer couples. As CBT for people with dementia and co-morbid depression has developed, it has become established that therapy can be adapted in various ways to allow for the memory and concentration difficulties experienced by these clients.

Charlesworth and Reichelt (2004) suggest that using shorter, more frequent and highly structured sessions which may be taped for review can make therapy accessible to those who are cognitively impaired, since the information provided is made more easy for them to comprehend and retain. Laidlaw *et al.* (2003) recommend the use of cue cards to remind clients of helpful cognitions and aid the process of cognitive re-structuring. Notebooks and index cards may also be useful for review of material and to keep track of homework assignments. The author has found that providing clients with a transcript containing a précis of each session, typed in large print for those with visual impairment, has generally been welcomed. Utilising a broad range of tools can therefore maximise a client's learning and potential for positive change.

A proper understanding of which abilities remain intact and which are impaired is crucial to doing this successfully. Laidlaw *et al.* (2003) point out that family members and carers can respond appropriately to disruptive behaviours if they are aware that these are due to the person's disorder rather than lack of concern for others. An accurate appraisal of the client's memory lapses can therefore ensure that realistic goals are set and productive interactions with others more likely to occur. The aim, after all, is to reduce depressive symptoms and optimise level of functioning.

Scholey and Woods (2003) reported outcomes and common themes from their CBT sessions with seven clients suffering from mild to moderate dementia (Mini Mental State Examination, MMSE 20–30) and depression. Sessions focused on clients' attributions about the cause of their cognitive impairment, often resulting in blame, anger and frustration, their catastrophic thoughts about the implications of the diagnosis, and the emergence of previous trauma. Only two clients showed a clinically significant improvement in their Geriatric Depression Scale (GDS) scores but the authors argued that:

> the cognitive shifts made by some of the participants and their descriptions and attributions of changes in their lives over the therapy period suggest that cognitive therapy did have some value… The therapist's perception from working with these participants was that they were slightly better able to accept their situation. They seemed to

be less confused and had better insight into their condition following therapy. (Scholey and Woods 2003, p.180)

The simplified formulations referred to earlier may take the form of a basic cognitive appraisal model consisting of the following sequence:

event ⟶ appraisal ⟶ emotional response

The term 'event' may refer to a range of experiences including life events, thoughts, emotions, physical sensations and the behaviour of others. Two- and three-element mini-cycles can also be used, as they are easier to understand than more complex cognitive models. These can then be elaborated upon as required. (For example, see Figure 8.1.)

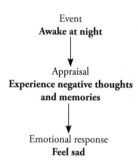

Figure 8.1 Cognitive appraisal model

CASE STUDIES

Roger

The following case study (Green 2007) illustrates how using such simple formulations and providing a summary of what had been discussed helped 'Roger', a fictionalised composite of various people who experienced depression following a diagnosis of dementia, to explore his difficulties. The interventions described are broadly representative of work done with these individuals.

Roger was an 81-year-old retired factory worker who had been diagnosed with Alzheimer's disease. His wife reported that he had been very low in mood over recent months and was reluctant to go out or engage in any meaningful activity. Upon exploration of these issues he revealed that he had lost his role in life due to no longer being able to drive or perform previously valued activities without assistance, such as gardening and decorating. Roger also acknowledged that he sometimes stopped doing things because he worried about his memory lapses being noticed by others. When he was asked to give a specific example of this, the formulation given in Figure 8.2 was arrived at.

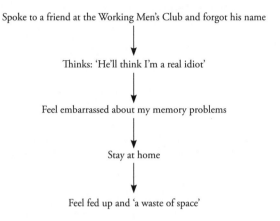

Figure 8.2 Roger formulation

SOLUTIONS

Roger's response was as follows:

- I would be sympathetic towards another person with memory problems.

- True friends will understand my memory problems and respect me for trying to lead a normal life.

- I participate in a reminiscence group at the day centre and have recalled my childhood, working life, holidays and hobbies. This encourages other group members to remember their own lives and they value my contribution.

- Continuing to go to the Working Men's Club, doing gardening with my wife and keeping active will help me to feel more positive about myself and feel better.

This particular example highlights how the experience of memory problems can trigger feelings of shame and embarrassment which result in a desire to prevent deficits from becoming apparent to others, leading to abandonment of activities and avoidance of social contact. Cognitions such as 'I am no good', 'I am a failure' and 'I am useless' are common, and the client typically believes that these thoughts will be shared by others. Consequently, the urge to hide, avoid exposure and run away predominates (Higginson 2006). The diagram in Figure 8.3 outlines how a compassionate mind approach, adapted by Higginson from the work of Gilbert (2005), can inform therapy when supporting individuals facing these difficulties.

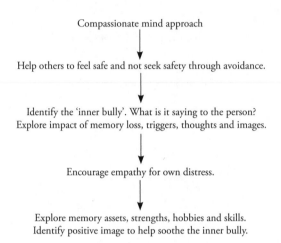

Figure 8.3 Compassionate mind approach

This approach was used to help Roger to challenge his negative perception of himself and make use of his abilities. Time was spent visiting him at home and accompanying him on walks in his local area and visits to shops and a café. He was surprised to discover that he did not get lost, could handle money and purchase items without becoming confused, and could enjoy pleasant conversations with friends and acquaintances. The benefits of doing this became apparent when, during one such outing, he found himself unable to remember the name of a fellow-member of his club whom he happened to meet in a café. Roger explained that he had memory difficulties due to Alzheimer's disease, asked the man his name and continued to hold a conversation with him. He did not experience any negative thoughts or feelings either at the time or following the encounter.

During one therapy session Roger was asked to imagine how he saw himself when he thought about not being able to do things. He responded by imagining that he was gardening and unable to perform the task properly. When asked how he would feel towards someone else in that situation, he said that he would 'feel sorry for him and want to help him'. Roger was then encouraged to feel as compassionate towards himself as he would towards another person, to imagine putting an arm around that image of himself struggling to do the gardening, and accept comfort and support. He found this soothing and was then asked to identify a more positive image of himself. Roger had spent many years in the RAF and was very proud of this, so he imagined himself wearing the medals he had been awarded. The following week he brought these medals with him to the day centre he attended and showed them to other clients and staff. Roger was subsequently able to identify a number of memory assets such as his wide general knowledge, ability to contribute to group activities, social skills and his recollections of all the places he had visited. He began to speak more openly about both his difficulties and his remaining abilities, remarking that his good physical health made him feel fortunate for a man of his age.

Sarah

Similar issues were explored with 'Sarah', a 78-year-old widow with Alzheimer's disease. (What follows is again a fictionalised composite, representative of the work done with several such clients.) She lived with her son, a travelling salesman who worked very long hours and was able to spend very little time at home with her. She had stopped going out, no longer participated in social activities and spent most of her time alone in her living room. Sarah reported that she frequently considered going out but would return to her seat before reaching the front door. The formulation in Figure 8.4 was arrived at after discussing this further.

SOLUTIONS
Sarah's response was as follows:

- When I went into town with my named nurse, I showed him where my favourite café was, ordered tea and toast and really enjoyed myself. I was able to find the correct change and hold a conversation with the girl at the till.

- I met four people I knew who were very friendly and obviously pleased to see me. They obviously don't mind about my memory problems.

- If I practise going out to places I know locally I will feel more confident and happy. Then I will not feel so lonely and isolated.

Sarah discovered that changing her behavioural pattern from one of isolation and withdrawal to one of meaningful activity resulted in an improvement in her mood and altered her pessimistic style of thinking. She was more significantly impaired than Roger and found it difficult to explore and challenge negative thoughts, but was able to retain information about behavioural change with the aid of a transcript.

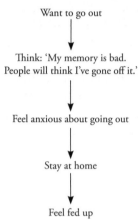

Figure 8.4 Sarah formulation

BEHAVIOURAL ACTIVATION

The development of behavioural activation (BA) as a stand-alone treatment, rather than simply a component of CBT, by Martell, Addis and Jacobson (2001) may offer a more appropriate intervention for moderately rather than mildly impaired clients. BA is a simpler and more parsimonious treatment than cognitive models and focuses on the idiographic context of the client's life. The emphasis is on behavioural patterns, how these are reinforced, what function they perform for the client and whether they result in the achievement of desired goals. Escape and avoidance behaviours may provide short-term relief in response to aversive life events, but are likely to maintain depression by creating secondary problems and denying access to alternative strategies. In BA thinking is conceptualised as behaviour, something we do, and the client is asked to consider the consequences rather than the content of what he or she thinks. It is therefore about the activation of the client rather than trying to change thoughts or beliefs.

Ekers, Richards and Gilbody (2008) conducted a systematic review and meta-analysis of behavioural treatments for depression compared to controls and other psychological interventions, concluding that BA was as effective as other recommended psychotherapies. Cuijpers, Van Straten and Warmerdam (2007) meta-analysed 16 studies of BA, finding large effect sizes in its favour, and the available evidence has been reviewed more recently by Sturmey (2009), who concluded that BA 'may be suitable for a number of populations and specific individuals who do not respond to CBT, such as people with poor verbal skills, those who are not psychologically minded and those who do not respond to cognitive or other therapies' (p.9). This simpler approach could provide an evidence-based alternative to cognitive models of depression for clients with dementia, perhaps combined with a compassionate mind focus, to encourage acceptance of negative thoughts and promote behavioural change.

There is some recent evidence to suggest that depression in people who are cognitively impaired is often characterised by motivational symptoms like loss of interest (Chopra *et al.* 2008) and that the relative preservation of procedural memories rather than language-based forms of recall provides a basis for behavioural interventions in therapy (James 2003). The relationship between dementia and depression is a complex one but recent research suggests that there is no particular association between the severity of cognitive impairment and the occurrence of depressive symptoms, which implies that intervention and prevention strategies should be aimed at all clients, irrespective of disease severity (Verkaik *et al.* 2007).

COPING WITH LOSS

Interactive theories posit a fluid connection between neurological and psychological factors, which may either reinforce or diminish one another, depending upon the specific situation of that individual, so depression can be both a risk factor for and a consequence of dementia (Alexopoulos 2003). This makes sense when one considers that the concept of loss lies at the heart of the experience of having dementia, in which 'cognitive and emotional decline interact in a cumulative fashion so that depression is aggravated by social and neurological changes; and that in turn, depression makes it harder for a person with dementia to withstand continued neurological deterioration' (Cheston and Bender 2003, p.154).

One can imagine the process of dementia as rather like holding water in cupped hands. Just as the water seeps away between the fingers, however tightly they are held together, so the person on this journey must see all that is remembered, even the very sense of self, slip slowly into oblivion. Therapy offers an opportunity to place another hand beneath those of the sufferer and help that person to retain for longer what they might otherwise lose more quickly than the natural disease process dictates. People with dementia face a future that is circumscribed, and any intervention which helps them to maximise their enjoyment of the present should be welcomed.

CODA

The tone of this chapter has been objective and scientific rather than personal, but I would like to end it with a story that illustrates the importance of supporting clients with therapeutic strategies which enable them to adjust to life with dementia.

Some years ago, I was involved in running a support group for carers of people with dementia. Reminiscence therapy sessions were run at the same time to allow carers to bring their relative with them to the venue if they wished. I clearly remember a man I will refer to as 'Jack' (again the description has been fictionalised) who had a relative attending the carers' group. He always seemed to be angry, joined in the reminiscence group for very brief periods and spent much of the time pacing the corridor outside. I was aware that Jack had been a freelance writer, and would sometimes try to engage him in conversation about his working life, but he dismissed my efforts as 'a waste of time'. My main impression was of an angry, embittered man who scowled a great deal, and I did not meet him again after the group ended, as he steadfastly refused to use any of our services.

About two years later I read Jack's obituary in a local newspaper. A picture emerged of an urbane, witty man who was the author of numerous books and the subject of many entertaining stories. The account of his life left me with a terrible feeling of sadness, since it was clear that his illness had robbed him not only of his abilities, but of his entire sense of being the person described in that article, of pride in his past achievements and acceptance of the person he had become. His barely suppressed rage had been a product of the unresolved frustration and despair which disfigured the closing years of his life.

Cognitive behavioural psychotherapy offers people with dementia, who struggle to cope with the losses they have experienced, the opportunity to adjust to their diagnosis, develop a realistic appraisal of their current abilities and overcome their sense of shame with self-focused compassion. The adaptations previously described can facilitate a clear understanding of the presenting problems on the part of both therapist and client, and support the retention of complex information. Further research is needed involving larger studies to make a convincing case to commissioners for the funding of increased CBT provision for this client group. However, the current evidence suggests that the inequality of access which still exists is completely unjustified.

CHAPTER 9

Gathering and Growing Gifts through Creative Expression and Playfulness

Susan McFadden

Annie, an elegant woman in her eighties, had advanced dementia and lived in a county nursing home. She rarely spoke and showed little interest in attending the many social events for residents. One day, three family members came to visit. The room was rather crowded, so her daughter and son-in-law sat on her bed, and her young adult granddaughter sat cross-legged on the floor. Suddenly, Annie picked up a small stuffed toy tiger and threw it to her granddaughter, who tossed it back. Then, Annie pretended to toss the tiger to her granddaughter, waving it at her and teasing her with it. Perplexed, her granddaughter burst out with a sound: 'Woof!' Annie laughed and threw her the tiger. Back and forth went the tiger, with the granddaughter 'woofing' and everyone laughing until they cried. Later, as the family left, Annie's daughter remarked that she could not remember the last time she had so much fun with her mother. About six months after Annie's death, the family gathered again to tell this story at a conference on dementia care. They wanted the audience of practitioners, family members, and persons with dementia to hear about how they experienced something holy in that afternoon with Annie.

Was this a really spiritual moment? The family interpreted it that way, but some people might say it was an undignified, childish interaction. However, if we understand spirituality as motivating humans to seek sacred meaning in relationship – with God, other people, the natural and human-created environment, and within the self – then we can affirm the family's experience as spiritual. Of course, this is not what people usually envision when they speak of such experiences. Calling this snapshot of silliness 'spiritual' is meant in no way to devalue grand 'mountaintop experiences' (which sometimes actually do occur on mountains) of the indwelling of the divine. Nevertheless, this family's play – wholly created by a woman whose dementia had robbed her of verbal language – transformed the moment by eliminating the distinctions between old and young, cognitively intact and cognitively challenged, male and female, and most any other differentiation human beings typically apply to themselves and other people. Using the language of Christianity, in that moment, these people were 'one in the Spirit' of God.

This chapter constructs a case for viewing creativity and play as expressions of spirituality understood as being grounded in the desire for a relationship with the sacred. After showing how this is possible, and briefly examining the reasons for resistance to this idea, the chapter turns to its core argument: honoring creativity and play can not only meet a spiritual need in persons with dementia, but can also nurture spiritual growth in those who participate in a 'new culture' of ministry with them.

They have much to teach us. As John Killick has written, dementia 'has the potential for enhancing our whole conception of what it is to be human' (2006, p.78). This is not a widely held idea, however, and too many people living with dementia lack the opportunity to nurture their spirituality in any way, including through creative and/or playful acts that help them experience their relation to the sacred. This situation should be unacceptable for persons of all faith traditions who profess the value of human beings without regard to age or cognitive capacity.

Any discussion of persons with dementia needs to recognize that, like all of us, they live in time. The expression of spiritual needs may evolve over the course of dementia and there may come a time when creative expression and play no longer function as meaningful ways of connecting with other persons and the realm of the holy. When this happens, spiritual care partners for people living with very severe memory loss need to call on their own creativity to infuse their shared time with meaning. This reflects the 'profound reciprocal influence of spirituality and interpersonal relationships' (Shults and Sandage 2006, p.161) implied by a relational view of spirituality. Although creative acts and play can both occur in solitude, viewing them as expressions of spirituality invites us to observe that even as forgetfulness and confusion advance, and death draws closer, meaningful relationships endure and other people can recall when their own spirits were touched by the creativity and playfulness of the frail person. In other words, Annie's family will long remember the day they played 'toss the tiger' together. Captured in that moment was Buber's relational vision of spirituality: 'Spirit is not in the I but between I and You. It is not like the blood that circulates in you but like the air in which you breathe' (Buber 1970, p.89).

CREATIVITY AND PLAYFULNESS AS EXPRESSIONS OF SPIRITUALITY

In the literature on the spiritual needs of older persons, we find many lists. For example, Harold Koenig (1994) described 14 spiritual needs, ranging from the need for meaning, purpose and hope, to the need to prepare for death and dying. All the needs Koenig cites are valid and important, and all reflect an appropriate sense of psychological seriousness, given the existential and spiritual challenges of aging. Later in his book, Koenig comments on the spiritual needs of persons with dementia and proposes techniques chaplains and clergy can employ in visitation and worship leadership. Koenig's suggestions are undeniably useful, but they do not invite us to consider how the human spirit might also be nurtured through creativity and playfulness.

In comparison, Albert Jewell's list of spiritual needs (2004, 2009) includes creativity as a spiritual need. Annie behaved creatively by engaging the family in pretend play as her granddaughter imitated a dog being trained to catch something. The outcomes of bringing something new into the world that has meaning – Gene Cohen's (2000) definition of creativity – can be 'severely practical or sublimely aesthetic' (Jewell 2004, p.19). We might situate Annie's creative solution to transforming an ordinary family visit into a spiritual experience as lying somewhere between the practical (e.g. making a new tool) and the sublime as expressed through various art forms.

Jewell (2009) notes that Jews, Christians, and Muslims view the human need to be creative as reflecting God's original creative force. Presenting his 'spiritual agenda' for older people, Jewell extends his discussion of creativity to include playfulness. Connecting play to creativity – an idea reaching back to Plato (Huizinga 1955) – and both to religiousness and spirituality can be problematic for some persons. Certain religious persons are suspicious of artists and their creativity (Wuthnow 2003) and may view play as a descent into idleness (called by some the 'Devil's pillow'). Christianity is well known for devaluing humour and suppressing laughter (McFadden 2004) through the work of 'a long line of grim theologians' (Berger 1997, p.198). However, psychologist of religion Paul Pruyser reminds us that to denigrate play eliminates recreation (re-creation) from creation. After all, says Pruyser, 'what can be more playful than a God who just speaks and things come into being?' (1968, p.253).

Play, laughter and humor, and creativity can all be seen as expressions of God's desire for human beings to enjoy creation with its many surprising juxtapositions and disparities that morph sometimes into comedy, and at other times into tragedy. The ever-present possibility that tragedy will ensue – a reflection of the essential vulnerability of human being – contributes to the deep pleasure of playfulness and comedy. After all, instead of leaving Annie's room feeling that they had experienced holy laughter, her family might have been overcome with grief that the elegant, sophisticated woman they once knew had deteriorated to the extent that she repeatedly threw a stuffed animal at her adult granddaughter. If they had accepted the predominant, one-dimensional image of memory loss as wholly tragic, then this family might not have been able to experience Annie's playfulness as a blessing.

Psychologists observe that the desire to bring something new and valuable into the world finds its earliest expression in children's play. As Erik Erikson (1977) noted, this creative playfulness is first experienced in the development of ritualized enjoyable interactions between infants and their parents. Erikson also observed that the first experience of the numinous occurs when infants gaze into the eyes of their mothers and fathers. Of course, the parents may not infuse this meeting with spiritual meaning, but those who do may perceive it as being sanctified. In the current language of the psychology of religion, sanctification is a 'psychological process through which aspects of life are perceived by people as having spiritual character and significance' (Mahoney et al. 2003, p.221; see also Pargament and Mahoney 2005). Annie's family sanctified their playful interaction with her; they felt God's presence in her room that afternoon.

Erikson (1977) believed that what begins in infancy as the ritualization of playful interactions between infants and parents becomes more formalized through the life-span as various rituals emerge to strengthen and grow relationships. Erikson recognized that ritual can take many forms, including the religious rituals of worship. Like other rituals, however, these can lose their meaning by becoming what he called 'ritualisms' – rigid, rule-bound, and drained of all creativity and playfulness.

Persons with dementia challenge ritualism. As any pastor knows who has ever led worship in a dementia care residence, people with memory loss can be quite uninhibited about interrupting a carefully constructed service.

This is one of the reasons family care partners sometimes hesitate to bring their loved ones to worship in congregational settings. However, rather than viewing their behaviors as frightening reflections of their neuropathology, we might see them as contributing to the drama of worship in their own unique ways. Their playful comments, vocalizations, and gestures remind us of the limitation of defining humans only as *homo sapiens*. As Johan Huizinga (1955) famously declared, we should not only describe humans as those who reason, and those who make (*homo faber*), but we should also include the important observation that all human culture involves the play of *homo ludens*. This can be amply observed in religious ritual, for, as Pruyser notes, 'religious behavior is full of playful features' (1968, p.191). The act of worship recruits human acts of imagination. We know that people living with dementia retain the ability to express themselves through imaginative creative acts (McFadden and Basting 2010; McFadden, Frank and Dysert 2008), and knowing this can point us toward a 'new culture' (Kitwood 1997a) of ministry with frail elders that embraces creative expression and playfulness.

A 'NEW CULTURE' OF MINISTRY WITH PERSONS LIVING WITH DEMENTIA

In his book *Dementia Reconsidered: The Person Comes First*, Tom Kitwood (1997a) described two cultures of dementia care and provided a succinct table contrasting the old and new cultures (see p.136). Kitwood was calling for a radical transformation of geriatric care as it had evolved primarily in institutions shaped by biomedical values. In opposition to this model, Kitwood wrote:

> The new culture does not pathologize people who have dementia, viewing them as the bearers of a ghastly disease. Nor does it reduce them to the simplistic categories of some ready-made structural scheme, such as a stage theory of mental decline. The new culture brings into focus the uniqueness of each person, respectful of what they have endured. It reinstates the emotions as the well-spring of human life, and enjoys the fact that we are embodied beings. It emphasizes the fact that our existence is essentially social. (Kitwood 1997a, p.135)

A new culture of ministry with persons with dementia is taking shape around the world. It embraces a relational perspective on spirituality and acknowledges the vulnerability and dependency of all persons, regardless of their cognitive fitness. This new culture affirms with Shamy (2003) that the denial of worship to people with dementia is a 'grave scandal' (p.95) and a 'denial of basic justice' (p.23). The new culture recognizes that it is unjust to claim to be offering an opportunity for worship to nursing home residents merely by scheduling a service led by a parish clergyperson (and listed on a daily calendar with other 'activities' like bingo) in a dining room lacking any signifiers that this is a holy place and time. This form of worship is often interrupted by clanging food carts and scented not with sweet incense but the odors of over-cooked meats and vegetables.

Thinking about transforming the culture of ministry with persons with dementia not only offers new perspectives for worship in long-term care residences, but can also point toward new approaches to congregational worship. In addition, it provides a model for congregational spiritual care programs for persons living with dementia and their care partners. When shaped by the old culture, these programs tend to reinforce passivity and victimhood. However, they can be transformed through an infusion of creativity and play.

INCLUSIVE CONGREGATIONAL WORSHIP

Congregational worship can be enriched by the contributions of persons with dementia, but doing this requires that worship leaders engage in their own creativity to come up with ways for persons with dementia to experience meaningful participation. These will vary according to the faith traditions of the congregation; the suggestions offered here may not be appropriate in some settings. In addition, worship leaders need to be sensitive to individual differences and the changes that occur with a progressive condition. For example, early in the journey of dementia, a worshipper might participate by reading scripture with a friend standing alongside to help keep track of the place in the text. Persons in the pews need to be educated in the inclusion of persons with disabilities, so that if a mistake is made, they will not be disturbed or critical but rather will celebrate both the courage of someone who still desires a meaningful role in worship and the creativity of the ones who helped to make that happen.

Musical talents are often preserved for a long time in dementia, meaning that individuals with these gifts can contribute through playing instruments or singing in a choir. In an article on music and the brain, neurologist Oliver Sacks wrote about the preservation of musical memory. For many religious persons, this musical memory would include beloved sacred music and hymns. Describing their experience, Sacks said:

> Familiar music acts as a sort of Proustian mnemonic, eliciting emotions and associations that had been long forgotten, giving the patient access once again to moods and memories, thoughts, and worlds that seemingly had been completely lost. (Sacks 1998, pp.11–12)

In the film *Young@Heart*, a 2008 British documentary about a chorus of older persons in Massachusetts preparing for a big concert, we see that one of the members of the 22-member group is experiencing memory loss. Nevertheless, the group continues to include him, and together with his family and the wider community, they celebrate his triumph in singing a solo. How many congregational choirs include persons with dementia, perhaps without even realizing it, especially with the current emphasis on early diagnosis?

The growing emphasis on the arts and creative expression as ways of offering meaningful expression and strengthening social bonds for persons with dementia (McFadden and Basting 2010) should inspire people thinking about a new culture of ministry to develop ways to integrate the arts and creativity into shared spiritual life. For example, mosaics, paintings, murals, collages, or other forms of visual art made by people with dementia could be displayed for the enjoyment and enlightenment of the whole worshipping community.

INCLUSIVE WORSHIP IN LONG-TERM CARE
As depicted earlier, worship in long-term care settings can be devoid of anything that nurtures the human spirit. But it does not have to be that way. Inclusive worship in nursing homes and other kinds of residences for persons with dementia means that children, teenagers, and adults of all ages mix among residents, singing, praying, listening, loving, and experiencing together the fact that 'religious behavior is full of playful features' (Pruyser 1968, p.191). Worship recruits faithful imagination, and even if people with dementia can no longer verbally articulate the stories about themselves as God's beloved that are woven into most worship experiences, they can usually still enjoy the various cues that they are in the midst of a loving, joyful community.

Sometimes long-term care residences have their own choirs of persons with dementia and even if a person can no longer verbalize a song, a rhythm instrument can be placed in a hand so as not to preclude participation. Psalm 100 invites everyone to make a joyful noise to the Lord and serve him with gladness. People with dementia holding rhythm instruments can make that joyful noise, and the children and teens present can participate too. Together, they can experience the spiritual uplift that comes with playful, creative expression.

Congregations in the community sometimes have liturgical dance groups; why should nursing homes be any different? Huizinga wrote: 'If in everything that pertains to music we find ourselves within the play-sphere, the same is true in even higher degree of music's twin-sister, the dance' (1955, p.164). People can dance in wheelchairs; moving in time with music, they can wave brightly colored cloths, all the while with joy celebrating the gift of embodiment that responds emotionally to music. A study of dance among people with dementia observed that 'participants seemed to forget their frail physical condition and minimal fitness level while dancing' (Palo-Bengtsson and Ekman 2002, p.151). Some Christian congregations sing a hymn called 'Lord of the Dance' that includes this chorus:

> Dance, then, wherever you may be;
> I am the Lord of the Dance, said he,
> And I'll lead you all wherever you may be,
> And I'll lead you all in the dance, said he.
>
> (Carter 1963)

This song says nothing about dance being reserved only for people who are young and fit – cognitively and physically.

CONGREGATIONAL SPIRITUAL CARE PROGRAMS
The old culture of ministry with persons with dementia is limited primarily to home visits by clergy and lay persons, not all of whom understand the intricacies of communication with a person living with memory loss and confusion. In the old culture, 'senior programming' for groups (which most likely include persons with dementia, whether diagnosed or not) consists of rather passive entertainment, often associated with a meal.

The new culture of ministry would nurture the spark of creativity and playfulness in all persons, and it would do it in such a way as to strengthen community, give people a valued social role (e.g. as one who creates, or actively participates), and offer opportunities for communication beyond words. It would celebrate the 'spirituality of the senses' (King 2004, p.138) in multiple creative ways. For example, instead of lining people up in rows to listen to someone talk about their 'trip to the Holy Land,' a program could be created to have participants gather around tables to paint their visions of the colors of ancient Israel. Herbs mentioned in the Bible could be passed round, sniffed, and tasted; much joyful noise could be made and people could imagine and show how David might have danced if he was in his eighties. As with other creative expression programs developed for persons with dementia (Basting 2008), these congregationally sponsored programs should include intentional rituals of greeting and parting. People working in secular programs for elders sometimes have trouble grasping the significance of ritualization of human interactions, but people designing new culture ministries ought to understand this easily.

Some congregations are collaborating to provide adult day programming and respite care (e.g. Brock 2008) where the creativity and playfulness of elders with dementia are honored and nurtured. If supporting an ongoing program exceeds the resources of a congregation, a new culture of ministry program might be designed around taking small groups of persons with dementia and their care partners to local art museums. The Museum of Modern Art's 'Meet Me at MOMA' program[1] offers a wonderful example of how people with dementia can enjoy programs that combine active engagement with great art, along with opportunities to create their own art works. The group might not even have to travel, as many religious congregations are blessed with artworks within their own buildings. Imagine, for example, a gathering of persons with dementia to observe and discuss the stained glass of a church or synagogue, followed by a time of creating artworks with colored glass.

WITNESSING TO THE WIDER COMMUNITY

In addition to stimulating new thinking about worship and congregational care programs, another goal for the new culture of ministry with persons with dementia should be to tell a story about dementia that counters the tale of suffering and loss most familiar to the public. When people with the diagnosis live in an environment that tends to the needs of the whole person – including spiritual need – spiritual growth is possible for them and those who love them. Witnessing to this possibility can take many forms. For example, congregations that promote creative expression programs could sponsor exhibitions of the works of persons with dementia as a way of giving them a voice in their communities. As Killick (Craig and Killick 2004) reminds us, their art should never be treated paternalistically. Rather, it should be honored for its expression of their agency in making it and their skill at communicating with those who view their creations. In this way, congregations could advocate for a different vision of people diagnosed with dementia, one that acknowledges the vulnerability of all persons regardless of cognitive status, and encourages the strengthening of communities where everyone has the opportunity to realize and grow their spiritual gifts.

LEARNING AND GROWING WITH PERSONS WITH DEMENTIA

By encouraging and supporting the creative expression and playfulness of people with progressive forgetfulness, and by entering into the 'now' with them (McFadden *et al.* 2008), we can experience what Houston Smith describes as the Taoist idea of 'life in tune with the universe' (1958, p.204): *wu wei*. Smith renders this as 'creative quietude'. It combines 'supreme activity and supreme relaxation' (p.204) and, when experienced, it can enable a person to arrive at genuine creation. Writing about the creation of art, Smith said:

> Genuine creation, as every artist has discovered, comes when the more abundant resources of the subliminal self are somehow released. But for this to happen, a certain dissociation from the surface self is needed. The conscious mind must relax, stop standing in its own light, let go. (p.204)

This can happen in our relationships with persons with dementia. Because their conscious, critical mind may be silenced, they can, as Thomas Merton (1961) wrote, 'meditate on paper' (p.216) and they are freed to play.

Working with persons with dementia to enable them to express themselves through creativity and playfulness, we are, as Merton says, planting 'seeds of contemplation' (p.14) in ourselves and in them. This may help us to understand that:

> What is serious to men is often very trivial in the sight of God. What in God might appear to us as 'play' is perhaps what He Himself takes most seriously. At any rate, the Lord plays and diverts Himself in the garden of His creation, and if we could let go of our own obsession with what we think is the meaning of it all, we might be able to hear His call and follow Him in His mysterious, cosmic dance. (Merton 1961, p.296)

When we enter into the 'now' moment with persons with dementia – persons like Annie who have lost self-consciousness and have stopped standing in their own light – 'we are invited to forget ourselves on purpose, cast our awful solemnity to the winds and join in the general dance' (Merton 1961, p.297) of life.

NOTE

1.   For further information see www.moma.org

CHAPTER 10

The Holistic Care of Older People in Care Homes

Gaynor Hammond

INTRODUCTION

Life is a mystery and it is amazing how our experiences, however seemingly insignificant at the time, can take us on journeys that we could never have imagined even in our wildest dreams. My background is in nursing, a career that I enjoyed immensely for many years, but latterly three significant events happened that were to change the course of my life completely: I started a theology degree; the hospital where I was working was closed down; and I went to work in a care home where many people who had dementia lived. Those experiences caused me to reflect on where God was leading me and the answer became clear when I took up the post of Dementia Project Worker for 'Faith in Elderly People' in Leeds. My role was to look at the spiritual needs of people with dementia and their carers and at how these needs could be met both by the church and by health careworkers.

Subsequently, I have worked closely with Christian Council on Ageing, MHA Care Group (Methodist Homes for the Aged) and the chaplaincy departments of Leeds and Bradford Teaching Hospitals. Working collaboratively with members of those organisations, I produced a number of booklets on aspects of spirituality and dementia.[1] I have also worked with the Baptist Union of Great Britain on care of vulnerable adults and helped to produce a booklet, *Safe to Belong* (Hammond and Owen 2006). I am now an ordained Baptist minister and a regional tutor for Northern Baptist College in Manchester.

During my years as a nurse I became increasingly aware of the importance of holistic care for older people. Good quality care takes into account the physical, emotional and spiritual needs of the whole person, and while most caregivers are familiar with recognising, implementing and evaluating physical and emotional care, the spiritual aspect is more difficult to identify and assess; indeed, there is for some careworkers a reluctance to consider the area of spiritual need. If spirituality is given any consideration at all, it is thought to be the role of the chaplain or community religious leaders. However, this does not take into account the breadth of meaning of spirituality and spiritual needs.

We all have spiritual needs, as we are all more than just body and mind. Care can be delivered on a purely physical level, and how we give that care may penetrate a deeper emotional level and, even deeper still, a spiritual level. Spiritual wellbeing can be described as the 'good feeling' brought about by a life lived in relationship with family, friends, community, the natural world and God. If a person's spirituality is linked to their sense of identity, then a spiritual need is being met when a person feels encouraged to be their 'real inner self', despite the outward changes of ageing, increased physical and mental frailty.

This is what led Laraine Moffitt and me to write a booklet giving guidelines and suggestions for writing care plans specifically for spiritual care (Hammond and Moffitt 2000). The guidance given in that booklet was about cultivating an approach to providing care which weaves spiritual care into the whole of caregiving. Nine years after that booklet was published, the time came to re-write and develop some of its themes, which I have done in the form of a training manual for care homes (Hammond 2009).

This training manual looks at ways to address some of the issues arising where good quality care is *not* delivered. Some of the suggestions given may seem rather simplistic and obvious. However, this is not always the case with a careworker who has had little or no experience of caring for a frail older person and has not developed the ability to empathise with how that person may be feeling about the care – or lack of care – that is all too often meted out.

Modern care practice is ideally person-centred rather than task-orientated. However, that does not remove the need for attending to 'the tasks'. What follows are some examples from the training manual of daily tasks, issues and rituals and how they can be delivered with due consideration of the physical, emotional and spiritual needs of the person receiving care.

THROUGH THE DAY
Wake up and start the day
The first task for any caregiver is to wake a person up to start the day. This may sound simple enough, but there are various ways to wake someone up out of a sleep. The carer could burst noisily into the bedroom, put on the main light, pull the commode up to the bed (have you heard the noise that

they make?) and wake the person up, if they haven't woken up already, as they are put onto the commode! The carer would have attended to physical needs but where in that procedure is the consideration for the person's emotional and spiritual needs? It can usually help to understand people better if we try to put ourselves in their shoes. Perhaps the careworker needs to think about how they themselves like to be woken up and consider how much more important it is caringly to help the person with dementia to adjust to their surroundings before being dragged out of bed.

A better way, therefore, would be to approach the person gently and put on a softer bedside light; greet the person by name and say who you are, where they are and what time of day it is, in order to help the person you are waking to orientate themselves gently. By doing this, you would be considering the person's emotional needs.

The way we greet someone reinforces a person's sense of value. We are saying 'It's nice to see you this morning'. Another way the caregiver could do this would be by taking into account individual choice. Does the person like to see the outdoors? If so, would they like the curtains open so they can see the sunshine or rain (providing of course the bedroom is not overlooked)? The carer could point out the view, the weather and the outside world. In such ways we can take into account the person's spiritual needs.

There are other considerations that can be taken into account in the context of holistic care. Is the person being cared for a 'lark' or an 'owl'? In other words, are they livelier in the morning or in the evening? If the person being cared for is sleepy in the morning, would it be possible to let them have a lie-in and get another person up who longs to be out of bed and start the day?

These are simple things but they can make all the difference to the person's wellbeing and would mean so much to someone who has probably already lost a great deal of their independence.

One of the worst examples of 'care' that I have witnessed was with a man called 'Richard'.[2] He found it difficult to get off to sleep and could be lying awake until the early hours, but when the morning came he would be sound asleep. He was incontinent and every morning he would be abruptly woken out of his sleep by being dragged out of bed, sat on a commode and his wet clothes stripped off him. When he swore at the carers he was told they had to do it because he was 'dirty'. A carer needs to ask, how would that make me feel?

The suggestions put forward in the training manual avoid looking at spiritual and indeed emotional needs as an extra chore to be added to an already heavy workload, but rather as needing to be woven into the whole of caregiving. It is not that it is new, but that it matters so much.

Mealtimes

A carer can begin by asking:

- What do I enjoy most about eating a meal?
- What is my favourite eating place?
- What might put me off my food?

In a care home, mealtimes comprise tasks that come round at least three times a day. Each meal can become a chore to get over as quickly as possible or it can be turned into a pleasurable activity.

Eating is often about more than nutrition. Consider all the reasons why we have meals: necessary sustenance, companionship, conversation, family gatherings, romance, religious festivals and celebrations. So, providing three nutritious meals a day would be caring for people physically. How the meals are presented would help the emotional wellbeing of the people being cared for. This would involve taking care over table settings, allowing people to sit with their friends, offering well-presented meals and giving people choices of what they would like to eat. It would be taking into account people's likes and dislikes.

Recognising a spiritual dimension to a meal might involve observing special festivals and celebrations such as Christmas, Easter, harvest, Passover, Divali, birthdays or anniversaries. On such occasions the care home could consider having communal meals together with staff, or inviting family and friends. Another way would be to consider the importance of giving thanks. Many faiths give thanks to God before a meal, or thanks could simply be given for the farmers, the chef or the earth for providing the food that is eaten.

The examples above present an idyllic view of mealtimes as the highlight of the day, something to look forward to, to be enjoyed. However, this is not always the case. There are care homes whose staff do not understand the importance of mealtimes and the joyful experience they can be – perhaps especially for older people, including those with dementia.

One care home I am acquainted with has three very confused people who need individual help, so one of the carers needs to feed them, and during this process the individuals often dribble the food out of their mouths. The policy of the home is that there should be no discrimination, and so these people would be seated at the same tables as other residents who enjoyed their food and made mealtimes into a real occasion. However, a couple of those residents just could not cope with having to sit opposite someone dribbling food out of their mouth, as it made them feel sick, forcing them to leave the table without finishing their meal. That social time, which they had previously looked forward to so much, was consequently ruined for them.

This is a situation where staff needed to be more empathetic with those in their care. Their intentions had been good, in that they did not want to discriminate against those who could have difficulty eating; however, they had not given any thought to the people whose mealtimes were now ruined. Also, how would the people feel who had difficulty in eating, knowing that they were 'in view' of all the others? The questions that need to be asked therefore are:

- How would you feel in such a situation?
- What could be done to help everyone enjoy their meals?

SEXUALITY

It is acknowledged that sex is one of the four primary drives of human beings, along with thirst, hunger and avoidance of pain. It is a myth that older people are no longer interested in sex. We are all sexual creatures, and remain such, but what we do with that sexuality and how we choose to express it is another matter, and to most people this is very personal.

However, living with dementia, or indeed living in a communal space such as a care home, brings all kinds of private issues into the public domain. Because of the nature of dementia, and the lowering of inhibition that tends to come with the disease, people may reveal their most private thoughts, feelings and behaviours – including those relating to sex.

This may lead to situations which are embarrassing for those close to the person, for the staff and for other residents, but they may also be very confusing, distressing and frustrating for the individuals themselves – especially when they cannot understand why their behaviour is considered inappropriate.

This is a sensitive matter and it is not helpful or appropriate to tell the person concerned to 'stop being rude'. It is important to try to sort the problem out without causing emotional or spiritual distress. It may be a matter of finding something for the person to do, using diversion to prevent their behaviour causing distress to others. And there are a number of ways to relieve pent-up sexual tension. For example, taking exercise and other energetic activities can help reduce physical tension, as can masturbation – maybe they just need some privacy.

Sometimes, sexual desire can be confused with a need for closeness, touch, belonging, security, acceptance and warmth, or the need to feel prized by another person. Some people find that, if they can meet these other needs, their desire for sex is reduced. Lots of people can be deprived of touch. Some have had very few hugs and kisses for months or even years. Many older people have been deprived of body contact for a long time, and this may add to feelings of loneliness. The need for hugs has been described to me as 'Not just about feeling someone's body shape pressed against you but about the aching void between your arms.'

These are real issues that need to be addressed sensitively and alongside the person who is acting in a sexual manner, since there may be others who become distressed at this behaviour. It can be a minefield of emotions. A hospital chaplain told me of an incident in a care home involving a new resident she was visiting, an 86-year-old woman who had been single all her life. The chaplain found this lady distraught and crying out, saying, 'He had no clothes on – that thing!' So the chaplain went to talk to the staff to find out what had happened. They all laughed and said, 'It was only Charlie, he walks round naked in the night and sometimes he has erections.' The chaplain pointed out how distressed the lady was, only to be told that 'It was only Charlie, she was all right.' Obviously she wasn't all right and her need for comfort and reassurance had been ignored.

If something happens that causes such distress, feelings must be taken seriously and the person cared for with sensitivity. That person needs to know they are listened to and understood, and that every measure will be put in place to prevent it happening again.

I have written about the need to develop an approach to care that includes the emotional and spiritual needs of the person. What happens when someone has emotional distress is that it can block the chance of any spiritual uplift or experience. Those feelings of anxiety and distress may last a long time if not dealt with carefully.

PERSONAL HYGIENE

This comes under its own category in the training manual, though there are issues around sexuality when it comes to something as personal as bathing or being bathed by someone else. A bath can be a very pleasurable experience. It can be an oasis away from a crowded situation. It can be a time to relax, soak and enjoy the sensation of the water. A bath can also be an incredibly spiritual experience if we think about the many symbolisms around water. It is a symbol of purification in many religions. Water is used for baptism; some Christian denominations use a whole tank of water for baptism by full immersion! It is a symbol of spiritual cleansing. It can be seen as the source of new life.

On the other hand, it can be a symbol of terror and abuse. Think about the elderly woman who is being bathed by a male nurse. Obviously there are nurses and carers of both sexes who are equally competent and caring. However, some older women may be embarrassed by this situation and even become distressed.

'Brian', an 18-year-old male nurse, was about to bathe an elderly woman, 'Martha', and started to undress her. She began struggling and screaming and another member of staff came in and shouted at her: 'Martha, if you don't let Brian bath you then you won't have a bath.' She wouldn't let Brian bath her, so she didn't have a bath.

It is important to think about this. There are many reasons why a woman might be frightened of any intimate contact with a man. 'Elsie' had dementia and she loved to see members of her family when they came to visit her, except for one, her eldest son. When he came Elsie would become very fretful and shout at him to go away – which caused her son a lot of distress. The problem was that the son resembled her father, who had abused her when she was a child. Imagine how Elsie would feel if she saw a man coming towards her with no clothes on in the night – or being bathed by a male nurse.

RELIGIOUS PRACTICE

To a believer, religion can offer hope. Someone with dementia or any other debilitating illness may feel they are losing control over many areas of their life, and belief in God may be one of the few things they feel they have left. People who have been believers for many years have a faith that is built into their whole way of life and personhood.

Words of hymns and prayers may be recalled long after other speech has been forgotten. If there is no opportunity for older people to express their beliefs through hymns, scripture reading, prayer and reflection, then their last ray of hope is being taken away. If someone has a faith history, then it is important for that person's relationship with God to be nourished by prayer, worship, fellowship and pastoral care.

It is therefore helpful to find out as much as possible about each person's specific religious needs. For instance:

- Which church did you attend?

- Who was your minister? Do they know you are here? Would you like us to ask them to visit?

- Were you involved in church groups such as women's meetings, men's fellowship, Bible study or house fellowship group, or choir?

- Do you watch 'Songs of Praise'? What are your favourite hymns?

- Would you like someone to pray with you from time to time?

Similar questions could be asked of individuals of non-Christian faiths, either directly or in collaboration with family members. Which mosque, synagogue or temple do you attend? Do you need a special day or time of the week for prayer?

Sensitive staff members can:

- show awareness of religious needs and make sure that those needs are met

- have time set apart from the daily routine to reflect, worship and pray

- provide opportunity for people to reflect on and talk about the deeper things of life and death

- encourage and welcome religious leaders and lay people to visit.

A group of people from a church used to visit a local care home to take worship services with the people who had dementia. They became disheartened because the people were very confused and could not seem to enter into the worship. After a few sessions a chaplain went with them and realised immediately what was wrong. First, the residents were seated at tables that had been prepared for the next mealtime. Second, there was no visible sign that they were entering a service of worship. Sitting at a table prepared for food gave the confusing signal that dinner was on its way, not that a worship service was about to begin.

A few changes made the experience more meaningful and people were able to engage in worship. The clutter of daily living was cleared away. A table was set out using symbols such as candles, a cross and flowers. A CD of hymns was playing as people came in. These small changes made a big difference.

CREATIVITY

Much human fulfilment comes from continued creativity. The deep desire to make things, to fashion materials, words and ideas, to make music, to nurture gardens, seems to be built into human beings. A basic and continuing human spiritual need is to express our unique personhood creatively. Having the opportunity to be creative gives meaning and purpose to life; it encourages self-expression, pleasure and laughter. It promotes physical, emotional and spiritual wellbeing, improves our feelings about ourselves and gives a sense of achievement. It helps the days to pass more pleasurably.

Imagine what it would be like if you had to spend each day doing nothing, day after day, week in, week out, each day like the one before. Would you feel like you were living or merely existing?

It is important for carers to think about the people they are looking after. Are they as active and stimulated as they might be? Could any more be done to help them get more out of life?

Consider these three stories:

1. 'Arthur' had dementia and, as his short-term memory deteriorated, he could no longer care for himself living alone and went into a care home. There was no stimulation, he became very depressed and his condition deteriorated. His family moved him to another home where there was a good programme of activities. After two weeks his son went to visit and found him in the lounge playing the piano with a group round him singing some of the old songs. It had been many years since Arthur had played the piano, and his son said the change in him was remarkable. The stimulation had greatly improved his wellbeing and given him a new purpose in life.

2. Two carers enjoyed helping the less able residents to make cards or play bingo, but the residents quickly became disengaged with the activity. What was happening is an easy trap to fall into. The carers were the ones actively engaged and the people they were 'helping' became just spectators, lost interest and felt useless. The best way of caring is to find ways to help the person become as actively engaged as possible and only step in to help when absolutely necessary.

3. 'Joan' had loved cooking all her life but had dementia and would forget some vital ingredient, so the cake would be ruined and this would cause her distress. Her carer found a way of putting out all the ingredients she would need, measured and in order. He would then put the oven on a timer so they would know when the cake was ready. In this way Joan was able to continue the pastime that she loved.

CONCLUSION

There has been a mixture of emotions, often embarrassment and reticence, among many careworkers regarding the nature of spiritual needs of people in their care. One of the aims of the training manual is to make the whole issue of spirituality less of a mystery and help careworkers understand the nature of spiritual needs and how they may be met for each person in their care. However, it is hoped that careworkers will also recognise how much they are already achieving in this vital area of care and feel encouraged and validated.

Acknowledging the spiritual dimension within all care practice may make it easier for staff to justify why bathing a certain resident took longer today than usual – it may be that today the bathing met that person's need at the deepest level.

Spiritual care does not need to become an extra chore added to an already heavy workload. The hope is that careworkers will be able to cultivate an approach to providing care which weaves spiritual care throughout the whole of caregiving: caring for the whole person. Trying to meet people's spiritual needs is at the heart of all good caregiving. It is not that it is new, but that it matters so much.

NOTES

1. *The Friendship Club* (Hammond 1999), *The Memory Box* (Hammond 2000), *Wells of Life* (Hammond and Treetops 2004), *Frequently Asked Questions on Spirituality and Religion* (Airey, Hammond, Kent and Moffitt 2002), all published by Faith in Elderly People, Leeds.

2. The names used in this chapter are not those of real persons and the descriptions given are composite, based on my nursing experience.

CHAPTER 11

Making the Journey Together

Palliative Care of Persons with Dementia

Wendy Shiels

INTRODUCTION

My sisters and I cared for our mother in her home after she was diagnosed with Alzheimer's disease. When her condition deteriorated, we were faced with the reality of our inability to care for her ourselves and reluctantly placed her into residential care where she passed away just ten months later. The whole experience was sad, isolating and distressing for her and for us.

As a family we were united in actively attempting to ensure that, as she could not speak for herself, the things that were important to her would be addressed and put into place. This included her very real need for privacy, for no fuss, and for quiet surroundings. While living in her own home she had always disliked background noise, so consequently radio, music tapes and television were rarely switched on. However, in her new 'home', despite our many complaints, the noise from other people and the television, which seemed to be left permanently on in the communal areas, made her cranky and cross. It also accentuated her disabilities – her speech became less intelligible, she became angry easily and we often arrived to find her anxious and crying.

Despite explaining to staff about her need for quiet, and their assurance that she would not be forced to spend each day in a communal area, this did not eventuate, as well-meaning staff insisted she was 'at risk of becoming socially isolated'. The results were predictable, and she soon had the label 'difficult behaviours'. We were losing even more of our mother. Life was very difficult and very sad for all of us. It was almost with relief that she passed away with her family around her a few months later – in a noisy shared ward with only curtains around us for privacy.

Following her death, I made an effort to follow up some of the problems we had incurred while caring for our mother, to see whether the experiences that we had were typical. I worked as a volunteer with Alzheimer's Australia

Victoria and underwent training in several areas, including that of an advisor on their telephone helpline (a position I held for ten years), as a sessional educator (a paid position) and as a public speaker for the Association. In 2001, I was awarded a Churchill Fellowship, enabling me to travel overseas to look at the different types of care for people living with dementia.

On my return, I made a career change, and since then have been employed as a dementia and palliative care coordinator in a large aged care home in suburban Melbourne. With enlightened owners and enthusiastic, progressive management, I was encouraged to investigate and try to solve the problems involved in personalising care in a home where the needs of 100 individuals and their families needed to be addressed.

We made an effort to find out what it was that a person moving into care needed to ensure an easy transition into such an environment, taking into account and respecting the individual needs of each person and the expectations of their families. Discovering background information as early as possible was vital, as was documenting it well. It required a lot of time and effort on the part of those collecting the information, and relied heavily on the cooperation and understanding of all staff and family members.

We formed a dementia support group, which has been meeting on a monthly basis since then, to support, educate and, if necessary, advocate for the families of people living with us.

Staff, who were already under pressure of the day-to-day workload, were encouraged to seek additional education specific to people living with dementia. This was part of my job description and using the experience I had as a family carer, coupled with my training and new experiences, I endeavour to help all the staff – nursing, lifestyle, catering and cleaning – to see the person behind the disease, and to appreciate their capacity for maintaining a purposeful and meaningful life, even while in care.

Sometimes there were no family members or friends who could give us good background information, and if the new resident was unable to tell us themselves, then the task of ascertaining what they needed and wanted was almost insurmountable. Occasionally, despite good background information from families, the needs of the person when they were younger and what they needed now had changed. For example, we were told by a woman that her mother, who was about to be admitted, had always been an excellent homemaker and loved nothing better than cooking. So she was included in our weekly 'cooking group'. However, she did not willingly join in and then, after a couple of weeks, refused to attend. When questioned, she said she had had to cook for a family all her life and she was 'damned if she was going to keep cooking now that there was someone else to do it'.

When a person living in an aged care facility is in the latter stages of dementia and can no longer communicate verbally, their capacity to make their needs and feelings known becomes severely impaired, so that their wellbeing and the maintenance of their personhood can be at risk.

I had read about a program called dementia care mapping (DCM), which had the ability to help us recognise and respond to the physical and psychological needs of people living with dementia in a prompt and positive manner. It had the potential to help heighten staff awareness of the capacity for this group of people to experience significant wellbeing. DCM is an evaluation tool used to assess and measure the emotional wellbeing of people with dementia. It is based on person-centred care principles as developed by Tom Kitwood, a British social psychologist and his team from Bradford University, UK.

DCM records, assesses and evaluates the experiences of people with dementia in care settings and bypasses the need to communicate directly with the person, relying instead on observation. It works on the assumption that people with dementia indicate their wellbeing and ill-being if they are observed closely over periods of time by a trained person referred to as a 'mapper'.

By focusing for periods of time on a person, the 'mapper' is able to understand what is happening to or around the person that is either enhancing or detracting from their quality of life. I trained as a 'mapper' in 2002, and have used DCM extensively during activities, at mealtimes and at times when nothing is happening.

We have used mapping to investigate the reason for large amounts of food being returned to the kitchen. These results indicated that some people did not like who they were sitting with, the position of their table, the noise created by the TV in an adjoining room or the menu. These issues were all discussed with staff and addressed: all seemingly small grievances, but things that made a difference to an important part of the day.

Using DCM I conduct a resident satisfaction survey that sits alongside the annual 'regular' survey. This latter survey is completed by those who are able to, or, if not, a family member may do it on their behalf. As a large percentage of the 100 people who live with us have a diagnosis of dementia, they are unable to complete this themselves, and only a very few of their families attempt to complete the survey on their behalf. As the results of the 'regular' survey are used to create a 'continuous improvement' program, this effectively means that the views and opinions of the majority of the people living within the care home are excluded.

The DCM survey was specifically designed for people who had a diagnosis of dementia and who were unable to reliably communicate to us how they were feeling about what was happening to them and around them in everyday situations. The areas covered by these surveys were the dining experience, activities, leisure time and receiving personal care: all areas which make up most of a 24-hour day. Times when people were sleeping or receiving personal care in the privacy of their own room were excluded.

The survey mapping was carried out over many, many hours with a representative sample of people. Not ideal, as it would have been preferable to map all who fitted the criteria. However, time did not permit this and it was hoped that the findings and subsequent actions would be of benefit to all. This has proved to be so.

Results of the surveys were evaluated and discussed with staff, and areas where improvement was needed dissected and, if possible, addressed. Gaps in dementia-specific education were identified and, based on these findings, an education plan was formulated.

The results not only gave this group of people a voice but, by discussing the findings of many hours of mapping with care staff as a team, we were able to focus on what else might be needed to increase wellbeing, then to work out how this could be implemented and included in their care plans to enable them to live as far as possible according to their individual needs. Mapping on a regular basis ensured that what had been introduced was acceptable, appropriate and working well.

DCM continues to be used to ensure that, as each person's needs change because of their declining medical condition, there is a focus on the maintenance of each person's wellbeing to the very best of our ability. This could be as simple as a preference for a particular type of music; to be seated near a window to enable them to see out into the garden; to eat in privacy; or to be given the opportunity to be passive observers in activities.

MARY'S STORY[1]

'Mary', 94, had advanced dementia and was unable to weight-bear or to communicate verbally. Mary spent her days in a 'fall-out' chair, needing full assistance for all areas of daily living. In the three years she lived with us, she never had a visitor. We had little idea of her background, other than that she had lived for several years previously in a supported residential home in the country. Her affairs were managed by the state.

Every morning, Mary was taken into the communal lounge area where many other people like her were sitting facing the television. On most mornings she appeared to be relaxed and presumably absorbed in the daily dose of a morning chat show! However, after an hour or so Mary would try to get out of the chair, attempting to swing her legs over the edge and leaning forward precariously. After being told many, many times to sit back, she would become very restless and call out loudly, often upsetting the others around her. As nursing staff were busily attending to other residents, there was little time to attend to Mary other than telling her, time and time again, that she would fall if she got up, and to sit back and watch the television.

Mary was labelled as being 'difficult'. When it was suggested she be left in her room, this was dismissed as putting her at risk, since there would be no one to 'keep an eye on her' and, by leaving her alone in her room, she could become socially isolated. There were no family members or friends we could discuss this with, and we had little idea of what Mary's preferences were, or what was needed now to give her some joy and quality of life.

It was decided to 'map' Mary for several days at different times. The results were pretty predictable and showed that Mary was bored, uncomfortable and frustrated because she could not move around. She was distressed by what was happening around her, possibly because of the amount of movement and noise coming from the television, and from the movement of staff as they went about attending to others in the lounge. This was all too familiar to me.

Mary's agitation, noise and restlessness were her only means of communicating how distressing this time was for her, and how trapped she felt, being left in a chair for the greater part of each day. It was her only way of expressing a need to escape situations over which she had no control.

As a trial, it was decided that Mary would stay in her room in her chair in a position where she could see out the window into the garden and where she could be seen by anyone passing her door. Regular safety checks were to be made and, as her room was situated in a busy corridor which staff and visitors constantly used, someone would frequently pass her room and be able to observe her easily without being intrusive.

When Mary had arrived at our home, she came with few belongings other than her clothing and a box of music tapes and an old, temperamental tape player. We purchased a new player for her, and the person responsible for monitoring Mary's safety was required to change the tapes. This meant she had one-to-one contact with someone, even though only for a few minutes, on a regular basis. At mealtimes, Mary remained in her room with the music switched off. Volunteer carers assisted her to eat, then stayed for half an hour or so, chatting or reading to her from the daily newspaper or a magazine. On leaving they would put a tape back on. Mary's volunteers grew fond of her and often brought a small bunch of cut garden flowers with them. It was obvious Mary looked forward to the visits. Mary's eating improved, and staff reported that she appeared to be napping off and on through the day, she did not attempt to climb out of the chair, rarely called out and was not, in their opinion, 'at risk'.

Mary was encouraged to come out and join others when there was a concert or particular activities such as flower arranging and craft, and by once again using DCM we were able to evaluate these experiences for her and to show that she appeared to enjoy her time as a passive observer, watching and listening.

What interests did Mary have previously? Was she an active person? Where were her family? What was important to her? What were her beliefs and her needs? We never did find out – but we knew that solitude and quiet were important to her now as were music, times to reflect and the company of someone special to her. Mary slipped away quietly and peacefully one night. Many staff members and volunteers attended her funeral service where three of her favourite tapes were played.

END OF LIFE CARE

One area that was of concern for us was our lack of information as to how a person would like to be cared for in the final weeks and days of their lives. What would be important to them at this time? Did they want to spend this time with particular family members or friends? Did they want to be transferred to hospital? What were their religious and spiritual needs? Unfortunately, when it did come to this time it was usually too late to seek out this information from the persons themselves, and it was left to their families to make this decision for them, often at a time of great emotional stress as they faced the impending loss of someone they loved.

Ideally, to ensure wishes are carried out, this would have been discussed and planned, and if possible documented, well in advance and well before a crisis occurred. In reality this rarely occurred, as many found this topic too difficult to talk about.

Several years ago Millward[2] adopted a program called Respecting Patient Choices (RPC) that originated in Wisconsin, USA, and was taken up and trialled in Australia several years ago, Millward being one of the first residential aged care facilities to trial and then to use the program.

RPC gives people the opportunity to think about, to discuss and to document an advance care plan before it is needed. This program does not advocate or support euthanasia, which is illegal in Australia, but encourages the person to appoint someone to make medical decisions on their behalf should they become unable to do so themselves. What is of paramount important in all these instances is that it is the wishes of the person concerned that are reflected in the document – not necessarily what the family or friends want themselves.

This exercise can be a very positive one for family members and gives an opportunity for them to get together to talk about, and think about, any comments or discussions that may have taken place beforehand with the person. Not only is preferred medical treatment discussed, but how the person would like to spend this time, with whom and in what surroundings.

What the plan does, as well as documenting their wishes for end of life care, is to add to our understanding of that person. Once the document is completed, it is filed in the 'resident's history'. The document may be revisited and revoked or altered at any stage, and is reviewed annually.

Amy's story

'Amy' was born in country Victoria in 1914, one of eight children, all of whom predeceased her. Amy married and was widowed twice, her first husband dying in the Second World War and leaving her with three small children. She remarried and had two more children, all of whom were still living. Her second husband died at age 80. Amy suffered multiple health problems, including Alzheimer's disease.

Prior to moving into care, Amy lived near one of her daughters. Her family were all loving and supportive of her and she was rarely alone, as at least one family member visited daily, often with one or more of her many grandchildren and great-grandchildren, whom she adored. They loved visiting her and played happily in her room, in the corridor or out in the courtyard – occasionally a little one slept on her bed. They brought in many of their kindergarten or school artworks, which were displayed with pride on her walls. Amy's room was her home – and theirs too.

Amy had been a very keen gardener and, after noticing the neglected garden in a courtyard outside her window, one of her daughters decided that under Amy's supervision, they would resurrect it. They contributed pots, potting soil and plants and spent many happy hours reviving this area. Birds nested in one of the pots and Amy ensured the birds had a water supply and seed. One bird built a nest in a pot right outside Amy's window and she spent many happy hours watching the mother bird sitting on eggs, then feeding and caring for two baby birds. There were many photographs taken during those nesting and hatching weeks, with Amy overseeing this with maternal care.

By choice, she spent most of her time (other than gardening) in her room surrounded by her family or staff. She ate (by choice) all her meals in her room, occasionally enjoying a beer, which she kept in a fridge in her room. The observation was made that this was probably the only stage in her life when she had been able to eat in peace and quiet. She had been a keen reader and, although unable to read now, still had a shelf full of books ranging from the romance novels she had loved to children's books catering for many ages.

She was a professed 'lapsed Roman Catholic' and, at the suggestion of her family, the visiting Roman Catholic priest called in to see Amy on his weekly visits, when she received communion. She appeared to derive much pleasure from something that had apparently been an important part of her early life.

Amy had no documented end of life wishes; however, over the years she had made it very clear to her medical practitioner and to her family that she was ready to 'go', and that her family should 'let her go' when the time came. She had said she did not want to go to hospital, or to have any aggressive treatment, and fortunately her family had talked about this and agreed that when 'the time came', she would stay with us.

Amy's heart began to fail and she was confined to bed. When her doctor suspected this might be her terminal phase, her family were invited to attend a meeting where her condition was discussed and a plan of care suggested. We were able to ensure her pain was kept under control, and she was kept as comfortable as possible. The priest visited and administered final prayers to her.

Amy's bed was moved right up to the window overlooking the courtyard and, despite her slipping into a deep sleep from which she did not waken, we ensured vases of fresh flowers were kept in her room where she could smell them.

Her family members drew up a roster which ensured that at least two of them were with her, assisting (by choice) with her care 24 hours a day. Amy was read to, talked to and held, and small children played around her bed. There were a few tears from time to time as different family members spoke about times during their Mother, Nan and Great Nan's life. When necessary they were comforted and supported by care staff and the palliative care team.[3] Meals and sandwiches were provided by us as necessary, and a bed and shower offered to anyone who needed to rest or to freshen up.

Amy passed away peacefully two days before Christmas with her many family members around her and with sparkly tinsel in her hair – a present from one of the great-grandchildren. Her funeral was attended by many of the staff. As in her life, the funeral service was anything but a sombre occasion, with young children participating in the service. Following her death, Amy's family donated her large collection of books to the home in her memory.

CONCLUSION

In an ideal world we would all die quickly and peacefully in our own homes, surrounded by those who love us. Sadly, this rarely happens when a person is living with dementia, with many families feeling as though they have 'lost' their loved one long before they actually die. However, with enlightened and educated carers, and programs such as Dementia Care Mapping and Respecting Patient Choices, we can ensure that to the best of our ability the personhood and abilities of this group of people can be identified and maintained.

When death is imminent, and particularly if there has been some dissension with the family, working together to ensure that the wishes of their loved one are carried out can often provide the opportunity to bring them together again and to enable them to move on in the knowledge that this was a happy release for someone who had led a long and fruitful life – a time to put aside past differences, to remember the good times, and to grieve together.

NOTES

1. In the case of both 'Mary' and 'Amy', names and situations described have been altered to ensure that privacy and confidentiality are preserved.

2. Millward is a 100-bed aged care home in Melbourne, Australia, which has embraced person-centred care using DCM and RPC. Its palliative care program is funded by donations received from the families of people who have been part of the program and is administered by a committee comprising representatives from the nursing and lifestyle staff, family members and volunteers.

3. Full definition of palliative care in accordance with the World Health Organization:

> Palliative care is an approach that improves the quality of life of patients and their families facing the problems associated with life-threatening illness, through the prevention and relief of suffering by means of early identification and impeccable assessment and treatment of pain and other problems, physical, psychological and spiritual. Palliative care:
>
> - provides relief from pain and other distressing symptoms
> - affirms life and regards dying as a normal process
> - intends neither to hasten nor postpone death
> - integrates the psychological and spiritual aspects of patient care
> - offers a support system to help patients live as actively as possible until death
> - offers a support system to help the family cope during the patient's illness and in their own bereavement
> - uses a team approach to address the needs of patients and their families, including bereavement counselling, if indicated
> - will enhance the quality of life, and may also positively influence the course of illness
> - is applicable early in the course of illness, in conjunction with other therapies that are intended to prolong life, such as chemotherapy or radiation therapy, and includes those investigations needed to better understand and manage distressing clinical complications.
>
> (World Health Organization 2010)

CHAPTER 12

Loving Attention

Chaplaincy as a Model of Spiritual Care for those with Dementia

Margaret Goodall

SETTING THE SCENE

The provision of 'spiritual care' for people living with dementia of all faiths and none has been a great challenge for those involved in delivering it. Questions are often asked about the nature of spiritual care, how it can be delivered and who should take responsibility for it. My context is working within MHA (Methodist Homes for the Aged), which has a Christian ethos. Chaplains are appointed in all our care homes and sheltered housing schemes as the focus for spiritual care, to work with care staff so that the needs of the whole person are met. Working effectively with those with dementia is a challenge, especially so in offering spiritual care, but reflecting on MHA's experience of chaplaincy this chapter is offered as a model of how it might be possible.

THE CHAPLAIN

The qualities we look for in a chaplain are genuineness and empathy – someone who can be alongside people; visit; give consolation; conduct services; offer the love of Christ and care for the spiritual needs of people of all faiths or none.

Campbell writes that it is, 'in essence, surprisingly simple. It has one fundamental aim: to help people to know love, both as something to be received and as something to give' (1985, p.1). This approach focuses on the 'kind of person the pastor has become rather than on her professional knowledge, expertise and skills' (Pattison 1988, p.141). Pattison also suggests that one pastoral skill that is lacking today is the ability to stand still for long enough for people to be able to know the pastor (1988, p.14):

> A being there, or loitering with intent or focus, is important in offering care. What is needed is someone who is not rushing, but able to stop and be open to seeing the world through their eyes and follow their story.

Asked how she would begin to meet the spiritual needs of people, one MHA chaplain answered, 'I would let them get to know me.' It is sometimes easier to keep a distance, to see 'us and them'. But to be truly alongside people who may be in distress asks that we are able to face the chaos and abyss in that person (Žižek 2006). To mediate care through being known suggests a relationship that is 'I–Thou' (Buber 1958).

Sheila Cassidy was involved in caring for people who, in worldly terms, are seen as beyond hope. She says that it is:

> a lavishing of precious resources, our precious ointment, on the handicapped, the insane, the rejected and the dying, that most clearly reveals the love of Christ in our times. It is this gratuitous caring, this unilateral declaration of love, which proclaims the gospel. (Cassidy 1988, p.2)

Goldsmith argues that dementia is 'another form of poverty, of powerlessness and of alienation' (1999, p.127), and that those who work with such people are on the frontiers of mission, responding to the passage in Matthew's gospel (25:14–30): 'In as much as you did it for the least, you did it for me.'

The chaplain is there for this way of relating: as someone who can reflect on the person's needs and offer appropriate spiritual care when the person cannot find it themselves. Thus doing, they enable others to see the difference it makes to the wellbeing of the person.

By employing a chaplain the aim is to have someone able to take this care seriously and be the focus of spiritual care. In MHA the post of chaplain is open to lay or ordained, of any denomination (with due training), and it is made clear from the start that the person appointed is to be there for all those in the home: residents, families and staff.

People come from diverse backgrounds and while, at present, most still have some religious affiliation or memory of church, an open approach to this ministry is necessary as people's belief systems become more diverse.

There are no conditions regarding belief attached to working in, or entry to, an MHA home, so this means that people of all faiths, and none, are to be supported in their spiritual life. We are still learning what this means but we state that all are to be respected, and that includes valuing what is important for them; so a Protestant chaplain could have a collection of artefacts from other faiths to enable residents to cue in to their faith, or remind them of the rituals for holy days and festivals. There is more to being a chaplain than celebrating Christmas and Easter. Indeed, MHA is in the process of establishing a multi-faith housing with care scheme in south Leeds, in which chaplains from various faith communities are to be appointed.

THE CHAPLAIN AS A MODEL FOR CARING

It is all too easy to view the chaplain in a purely functional role: conducting a service, or taking tea with people. The observant may have seen individuals encouraged or comforted by talking or simply being with the chaplain. However, it is the one-to-one time with people that is at the heart of spiritual care. Staff involved in the day-to-day care necessarily have their attention on immediate concerns, but the chaplain is a model for those who can give time and attention to the person. What residents crave more than almost anything else is someone who will be there for them. When asked what they want from carers, older people have said, 'someone who knows me'. One person cannot deliver all the spiritual care a person needs, but the chaplain is a reminder that spiritual care is at the heart of all care as it affects the whole of life.

There is a need for someone to be responsible and accountable for spiritual care because it demands attention at a deep level. While all in care roles will in some way be offering spiritual care, it needs someone to hold all the experience of God and people together and make this accessible. The whole of life, death and everything in between is encountered in the care home, and while traditionally this role has been associated with the clergy there is no reason why, with support, a lay person cannot do this. What *is* important is the ability to be open, to make relationships and to reflect. Spiritual care should be informed by many voices and the person offering such care should be willing to experience a powerlessness and vulnerability, not seen as someone who 'has all the answers'.

The following comments show the range of reflections and concerns that MHA chaplains have raised related to their role.

- 'I have health problems but the residents like my vulnerability. They say that it's usually "us and them" but we can minister to you. I seem to have brought Christ into an unlikely place.'

- 'Is being a chaplain more than just chatting to people?'

- 'How do I recognise when I am listening to others and when I am chatting for the sake of it?'

- When the group learnt that 'N' was doing exercise classes for residents, one chaplain asked, 'Where does the line come between doing activities and chaplaincy?'

- 'How can we lead worship when most are asleep? What kind of spirituality is this?'

- 'Working with the activity co-ordinator is good. It's more risky on your own.'

- 'I've learnt that you can't do things quickly. I have to slow down and take the moment.'

- 'What I value is the look that tells me I've reached somewhere in someone.'

- 'The home has been through a period in which we've experienced a lot of deaths in a short space of time. There has been a distinctive role for me to play alongside other staff in supporting families through times of bereavement and being involved in funerals.'

- 'Relationships changed for the better in the home after the staff came to a funeral that I conducted. It was as if they saw me as being able to do something they couldn't. They appreciated the knowledge I had of the person and they felt I honoured his life.'

- 'It's important that I am able just to pop in. I belong and am seen as part of the furniture and have my own mug for tea!'

What becomes evident from these comments is that chaplains are aware that they are in a place that does not fit comfortably with usual structures, and that they have to earn their place as a part of the staff team. The comfortable place can often be where they are 'doing' and being productive. But true chaplaincy is more about 'being', a 'loitering with intent', able to reflect and respond as needs are presented. The kind of 'helping' that they are engaged in can be in creating 'a space where people can come to know themselves and their situation better; to see possibilities and to believe that change is possible; and to take steps to overcoming something that is troubling or facing them' (Smith and Smith 2008, p.15).

SPIRITUAL CARE

Those with dementia are some of the most vulnerable in society, and good care should be more than the merely necessary as we care for the wellbeing of the whole person. Eileen Shamy argues that 'Neglect of the spiritual dimension of care seriously impoverishes the quality of life for people just as surely as neglect of the physical dimension – though the latter may be more apparent' (1997, p.55).

Using the word 'spiritual' can make some switch off and defer to someone from the church. But, to be holistic, care needs to include spirituality, as it is concerned with the whole person. When that person has dementia, then spiritual care should be offered, using best-practice of dementia care. This type of care comes from an understanding that is informed by a relationship with the person.

'Spirituality' is difficult to define, as it means both anything that gives meaning and purpose to life, and also what is found in following a faith. In secular terms it is anything beyond the merely material and seen as a way of making sense of life that may or may not have a religious basis. Spirituality is defined in the Age Awareness Project of MHA and the Christian Council on Ageing as: 'a quality that goes beyond religious affiliation; that strives for inspiration, reverence, awe, meaning and purpose, even in those who do not believe in any god' (Harris 1998, p.2). Talking about an inclusive spirituality has been difficult because many would only have come across the term when used in a religious context (Chatterjee 1989; Airey *et al.* 2002).

Reminding people of the culture that they belong to is an important part of affirming their identity and enhances their spirituality. Elizabeth MacKinlay suggests that 'Frail older people need the presence of familiar symbols, language and rituals to support their continuing identity' (2010, p.15). Religious symbols have always been important and convey layers of meaning beyond the symbol itself. For those with dementia, who can become increasingly isolated, to have their faith culture affirmed in the context of shared beliefs, values and liturgies would go a long way to supporting their spirituality and their autonomy. For those with no faith, meaning and purpose can be found in the rituals of our shared life; in family, art and nature. What is vital is to find out what gives meaning for the unique individual and discover the 'pearl' at the centre.

Good spiritual cares relies on awareness and reflection and needs to be searched for with intuition and imagination (Stanworth 2004). For those delivering care it could be as simple as recognising that all good care is spiritual care, since good care is person-centred care offered with sensitivity.

MEETING THE SPIRITUAL NEEDS OF SOMEONE WITH DEMENTIA

As a person's dementia advances, thinking becomes more concrete as the rational parts of the brain are lost. The world appears to be framed by the senses: by what can be touched, seen, heard, smelt and tasted. 'What if?' questions baffle and confuse and, even when speech is possible, people lose their capacity to initiate conversations or discuss abstract ideas (Goldsmith 1999).

It is argued that 'spiritual wellbeing becomes more important when physical and psychological decline occurs' (Harrington 2010a, p.180), so for those with dementia finding ways to encourage their spiritual life becomes increasingly important. If spiritual wellbeing is the affirmation of life in a relationship with God, self, community and the environment (Ellor, Stetner and Spath 1987), then good spiritual care taps into the feelings and the memories, which means that personhood is affirmed.

We have difficulty trying to envisage what people with dementia need, since their world can seem closed to us. But we now have books written by people who have dementia that have opened up their world to us (Davis 1992; Bryden 2005). These voices can give us clues about what it could mean to the person to offer religious and spiritual care. Christine Bryden writes through her own experience and, while each person's journey of dementia will be different, her writing gives us an insight into what, for the onlooker, can seem puzzling and beyond imagining. To those who suggest that in losing rational thought those with dementia become less human, she says:

> I believe that people with dementia are making an important journey from cognition through emotion into spirituality. I've begun to realise that what really remains throughout this journey is what is really important. (Bryden 2005, p.159)

In her writing she reminds us that for her and others like her, spirituality is:

> not simply what religion we practise; it is what has given us meaning in our lives. Our garden, art, pets, the familiar ritual of religion. It is important to help us to reconnect with what has given us meaning as we journey deeper into the centre of our being, into our spirit. (Bryden 2005, p.123)

Dementia has been associated with the loss of self, which implies that at some stage the person ceases to be human (Goldsmith 1999). This can cause stigma that threatens spiritual identity. Bryden (2005, p.152) suggests that 'this is silly... Exactly at what stage do I cease being me? My spiritual self is reflected in the divine and given meaning as a transcendent being.' If spirituality and identity are not diminished with dementia, then people continue to have spiritual needs that we have a responsibility to meet through our care, recognising that whatever happens, there is a core that remains oneself, a continuity of self (Mowat 2004).

The spiritual tasks of old age are not changed by dementia, just made more difficult for us to see. However, just as they need assistance in all areas of daily living, those with dementia find meaning, purpose and love through contact with others. When their spiritual needs are met, the result is seen in the quality of relationship.

RELATIONSHIP AND PERSON-CENTRED CARE

Most people find their deepest personal meaning in relationships, and those with dementia are no different. They are dependent for every need on those who know them, and the care received is only as good as the relationship between caregiver and care-receiver.

The basis of person-centred care (Kitwood and Bredin 1992b) is that the carer sees and responds to the person, not the presenting problem. This is demanding both of attention and intuition. If spiritual care is effective the carer will observe that the person is expressing a feeling of wellbeing, of being in control, or simply not feeling anxious about their care or their situation (Bryden 2005; Cobb 2005). People give cues, in both their actions and their emotional state, so inability to reason or answer questions should not be a bar to recognising the need for appropriate care. Christine Bryden says that is because those like her who have dementia 'live with a depth of spirituality...rather than cognition, [that] you can connect with us at a deep level through touch, eye contact, smiles' (2005, p.9).

One difficulty for chaplains, and others, is that they are not used to watching residents so attentively, or of recording the feelings and emotions observed. This requires time which people often do not have. Attention and then reflection are vital in assessing spiritual care, both in order to discern what is needed and then to evaluate. This method of care is intentional and a way of showing loving attention which is at the heart of good care, but this involves a cost to the caregiver. This is especially so when the emotional demands of such care are considered, and Harrington (2010a, p.188) suggests that this is one of the barriers to spiritual care.

THE 'FRUIT OF THE SPIRIT' AS A METHOD FOR OFFERING SPIRITUAL CARE

One way of assessing spiritual needs is by testing observed feelings and emotions against the qualities defined by the Biblical concept of the 'fruit of the spirit'. (The 'fruit' listed in Galatians 5 are: love, joy, peace, patience, kindness, goodness, gentleness, faithfulness and self-control.) These are not individual qualities but are rooted in the 'I–Thou' relationship (Buber 1958): our interaction with God and with others. Person-centred care is based on this idea of relationship, so this method could enhance the best model we have for care of those with dementia.

The work of the spirit is to breathe life, to enable relationships and to help us look outside our own needs and wants and feel for others, and it is in this working out of relationship that we find the 'fruit of the spirit' displayed. The life qualities found in 'fruit' show ways of relating to both the non-material and the specifics of faith, and can enhance the spirituality of both religious and secular people. Spirituality can thus be seen in the comfort, love and peace that individuals experience in their relationship with self, others, nature and the transcendent. This in turn can elicit a sense of being 'more at home' in the world (Macquarrie 1972) as those concerned experience a sense of connection and inner strength.

THE 3 RS OF SPIRITUAL CARE

In practice, using the 'fruit of the spirit' as a guide to spiritual care could be offered using the 3 Rs of spiritual care, which are: *reflection, relationship* and *restoration*. The chaplain/carer can give attention to the person and *reflect* on their mood and demeanour for signs of ill-being and what might be needed; through the *relationship* they have with the person discern some way to meet the need and offer appropriate care; and then recognise the *restoration* (change) in the person (Goodall 2009).

The 'fruit of the spirit' can be used to identify spiritual needs and then as a check through observation to see if the need has been met. For example, if someone *is* very restless, and all their physical needs have been met, then ill-being would seem to point to a lack of peace. By taking the person aside, listening and speaking gently to them, in a way appropriate to their beliefs (known because of the relationship that exists), this spiritual need may be met and they may find themselves in a different place with a sense of peace that was not there before.

Chaplains to dementia homes are aware that there is much trial and error, and 'gut feeling', in their work, but it is by reflecting on what care is and is not accepted by the resident that a way to meet their needs will be found. If others are able to observe this, then they too will be empowered to offer this care.

There is a wider application for the model suggested than just for those with dementia. If it is successful with this group of vulnerable people, then it can be offered as base-line spiritual care for all who find it difficult to communicate their needs.

LOVING ATTENTION

Spirituality is an important part of most people's lives, but while some experience spiritual moments in the everyday, for others it requires particular places, times or events. It is where people are not active, or no longer able to access help for themselves, that chaplains are often provided, especially when those people are also vulnerable or anxious. It can be difficult to visit a person with dementia, as the one visiting can feel de-skilled, and indeed the visit may at times seem mundane, but Christine Bryden gives this reflection:

> I treasure your visit as a 'now' experience in which I have connected spirit to spirit. I need you to affirm my identity and walk alongside me. I may not be able to affirm you…but you have brought connection to me, you have allowed the divine to work through you. (Bryden 2005, p.110)

At the heart of chaplaincy is a sensitivity to and an understanding of all kinds of relationship, the ability to reflect on what they see, ability to provide care and support for residents, their families and staff, and ability to work alongside other professionals. Chaplains do not work in isolation, and the best working will be through partnership between staff and chaplains that leads to a mutual understanding of the goals of spiritual care (Rhodes 2005).

If chaplains are to be seen as part of the team who offer care, then they also need to play their part in demonstrating good practice through evidence-based care (Folland 2005). This is a foreign concept to many, and for those who offer this chaplaincy alongside an already busy ministry, it may be one request too many. But if the work of chaplaincy is to be valued by others in the team, then it must offer the very best practice.

The South Yorkshire Strategic Health Authority's *Caring for the Spirit* report (2003) assumes that record-keeping is already part of the role and task of chaplaincy. Evidence-based care and the recording of such allows others involved to share in particular insights that will enable continuity of care that can only benefit the person being cared for.

Spiritual wellbeing has been recognised as an important part of holistic care since 1971, but has not always been evident. Perhaps one of the reasons is that, in order to assist individuals with their spiritual needs, the one offering the care needs to be attentive to their own spirituality. The chaplain is a model for what is possible when someone has the responsibility for spiritual care.

A visit from the chaplain is more than sharing a cup of tea, though that may be an important part of it. It is a focused meeting where loving attention is given to allow connection and the work of the spirit, the go-between God. We cannot answer the question 'Why?', especially when that relates to dementia. 'But we can, with careful attention, offer such care that meaning and integrity can be found and so enable the journey into a good death' (Goodall 2010, p.114).

CHAPTER 13

Resilience Promotion and its Relevance to the Personhood Needs of People with Dementia and other Brain Damage

Murray Lloyd

THE CHALLENGE

In my 30-year travels as a consultant physician in the fields of cardiology, rehabilitation, palliative care and, finally, aged care, I did my best to broaden the approach of my fellow clinicians with presentations and articles that reminded them that illnesses are contained in human beings. At the end of my career I realise what a difficult task I was undertaking. The key problems I have identified are very relevant to providing a better deal for the key focus of this chapter, the elderly confused. My hope is to prepare readers to be both patient and dogged as they are confronted by the barriers that exist to meeting the personhood needs of those for whom we have responsibility.

Highlighting the key elements of what I have learnt leads to the core concept of this chapter, namely that using the resilience promotion model can open up dialogues that facilitate better understanding of the need for very significant paradigm changes in our care style.

A major problem is that each helping profession has its own special language and approach, but a commonly held attitude, probably strongest in the medical profession, is that the areas defined by the words 'holistic' and 'spiritual' are not really part of clinical responsibility. The word 'spiritual' is often not well defined and is commonly translated as meaning religion.

In 1997 dementia trail-blazer Eileen Shamy (1997, p.54) wrote:

> Many New Zealanders of European descent, with the exception perhaps of those in touch with their Celtic origins and culture, are likely to be a little touchy about the word spiritual, confusing it with religious…[it] has been deliberately excluded and separated out from public life and confined to an individual's private life.

Psychiatrist Russell D'Souza (2002, p.S57) explained the problem with the medical profession:

> As doctors, we have been trained to be 'objective' and to keep our own beliefs and practices separate, but over time we have strayed into keeping the patients' beliefs, spiritual/religious needs and supports separate from their care. Thus, we are potentially ignoring an important element that may be at the core of the patients' coping and support systems and may be integral to their wellbeing and recovery – which is what we set out to achieve in the first place.

Thus, for clinicians of my era, religion and spirituality were seen as outside their domain – too sensitive, too dangerous, not clinical – definitely a taboo area.

The emotional response to 'holistic' was that this was all about crystals, communicating with the spirit world – and the complex and poorly understood field of 'complementary medicine'. The language of secular spirituality, with its practical connection to modern self-improvement programs such as cognitive behavioural therapy, was not recognized.

This chapter will illustrate the language that was developed in attempts to overcome this scepticism with a view to improvements at both administrative and staff levels.

KEY DEVELOPMENTS

In my years in formal aged care beginning in 1984 there were two key programs that paved the way for the changes in dementia management that were drastically needed.

The first was validation theory (Feil 1982): 'accepting people where they are'. The second is what we now know as the 'personhood approach' (Kitwood 1997a). This concept has developed particularly in the field of dementia but its importance extends very strongly into all chronic and life-threatening disease.

If medical administrators and planners do not recognise what they often think of as the 'soft' or 'mystical' side of care, this essential part of end of life management will not be properly funded. In general, this change cannot be expected to come easily and in secular Australia the going has been predictably tough.

A string of programs throughout my career have attempted to highlight and teach the importance of psychological security in illness. This has now been well documented in the isolation that occurs as part of all stages of the dementing process.

In 1970, discovering the three-sided triangle of the Greek bio-psycho-social model was the first wake-up call that my medical teaching had missed something. The basic idea was that if any one of the three sides of this triangle (physical, mental, social) was unhealthy, the health of the whole person suffered; their coping energy became depleted.

Antonowski (1987) promoted the concept of 'social coherence' and carried out assessments of the items that create this personal and social strength factor that is now widely used in sociology. One of his factors was the theme of Viktor Frankl, whose *Man's Search for Meaning* (1984) emphasis can be seen as a major advance in understanding what makes humankind tick, particularly in chaos situations and at the end of life.

In Australia, Caroline Jones' radio program 'The search for meaning' and her book (1989) provided a strong impetus to the idea that sharing personal inner dialogues and feelings is 'OK', as well as very productive. Howard Clinebell (1995, p.6) provided a model whose poetic definition shines through the fogginess of this terrain and links with the major advances in dementia care that were in progress:

> Wholeness, like a flower, is a living, growing, ever-changing unity among all its parts and with its environment. The centre of the flower stands for healthy spirituality. Such spirituality holds the petals of wholeness together and gives them organic unity. The centre is also where the petals are nourished and the seeds of new life grow. The roots of the wholeness flower go deep to draw nutrients from the soil of our common humanity and from the biosphere, the wonderful web of living things from which our food comes. The air with which the flower interacts surrounds it.
>
> Above the flower is the sun of Love – the divine source of healing and wholeness. This sun supplies the energy that enables the flower to continue to grow, stay beautiful, and, in due time, produce seed. Like the flower, wholeness has its seasons and its birth–life–death–rebirth cycles. There are times of seed planting and germination, blossoming and seed-making, withering and dying, returning to the earth – in preparation for the new generation in the cycle of continuing creation.

Placing 'spiritual' at the centre of the holistic model created a new model by splitting 'mental' into feelings (emotional) and thoughts (cognitive). The 'doughnut-shaped' model that resulted in my work (Figure 13.1) can be applied very neatly to an analysis of clinical situations such as dementia and depression (Lloyd 2003).

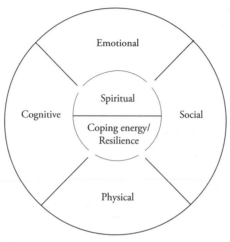

Figure 13.1 Holistic model

'Spiritual' (see Figure 13.1) has been placed at the core of what is now a deeper representation of the human being that is the full focus of care. Note that the horizontal line remains to represent the variable pool of coping energy that is later to be labelled as resilience. The vertical line is an indicator of the developing contemporary concept that there are two types of spirituality: religious and secular.

A clinical definition particularly derived from the Methodist MHA Care Group's program *Nourishing the Inner Being* (2002) was synthesised. It emphasised a pathway that clinicians could follow in relating more deeply to the needs of their patients.

Suggested clinical definition of spirituality

In an article in the *Journal of Dementia Care* (Lloyd 2004, p.25) I offered the following definition:

> Spirituality is the part of our life experience that is processed by the human spirit. The human spirit is the centre of energy whose core function is to give continuing meaning to our lives and nourishment to our inner being. By surveying and appraising our connections with the environment and in relationships, it creates a dialogue within ourselves through which we privately weigh up the meanings of deeper aspects of our life experience – visible and invisible – positive and negative – past, present and future. For many, a relationship with a life force represents a challenging part of this process.

An indicator of the climate I was working in was the comment made when I asked why a paper presenting this approach was turned down for a national conference on ageing and pastoral care. The reply to this cheeky 'why?' request was 'who did I think I was to be redefining spirituality when so many illustrious people before me had done this?'

Another example of this problem zone was shown in an Australian Commonwealth-funded program *Challenging Depression* (Fleming 2001). It covered many approaches that could be taken to prevent and manage the high incidence of depression and its often associated dementia in residential villages for older people. However, when the word 'spiritual' was approached the gap that existed was vividly shown. A huge area of important work was not even mentioned. The program had omitted all developments at the time that came under the heading of 'personhood validation'. The names Kitwood, Shamy, Killick, Goldsmith, Bright, MacKinlay and Frankl among others did not get a mention. Similarly, the two important training videotapes, 'One to One: Towards a Deeper Level of Communication' (Chapman and Killick 1997) and 'Nourishing the Inner Being' (MHA Care Group 2002), were not listed as resources.

It was clear that the word 'spirituality' was too awkward for this otherwise excellent team of consultants. This suggested that workers wanting to put into place 'spiritual enhancing' programs would run into a lack of administrative enthusiasm and funding. It was almost as if a Commonwealth-funded program could not risk the controversy of religion and its shadow, spirituality.

My article in reply, 'Challenging depression – taking a spiritually enhanced approach' (Lloyd 2003) centred on a holistic diagram of the origin and treatment of depression. It listed and summarised the many programs and approaches that could be very relevant to supply the particular need that the program's depression assessment process had identified. Under the heading of 'spiritually enhanced approach', the therapy opportunities listed around the holistic 'doughnut' were a long way from the dominant tablet-based approach using antidepressant and antidementia drugs. It is, of course, not possible to assess what impact this article had. A point to be noted is that important areas of work can be missed by experts when the topic is felt to be a mystical one, one in which it is difficult to establish an evidence base.

In my article in the *Journal of Dementia Care* (Lloyd 2004) 'Understanding spirituality: tuning in to the inner being', a reinforcing model was offered. It was based on Maslow's hierarchy of needs (1943): the hierarchy of elderly spiritual needs. Figure 13.2 illustrates the idea that the ultimate goal of hope, purpose and tranquillity cannot be reached until a basic foundation of security is there. The middle sector challenges carers to be more understanding and skilful in their engagement with older people, particularly when, as in dementia, there may be behaviour that is challenging and hard to understand.

The process labelled as 'spiritually enhanced active listening' was defined by suggesting that empathy of a deeper level can be expressed by phrases that identify with the basic feelings that give rise to emotional ones. An example from the video 'Responding to Music' (Mullan and Killick 2001) was used to describe the inspired guesswork that may sometimes lead to recognition of a transcendent experience from the past.

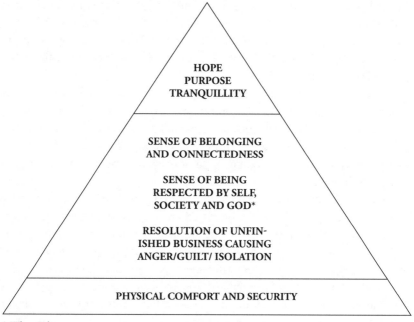

Where Relevant
Figure 13.2 Hierarchy of spiritual needs

RESILIENCE

Onto this scene a new concept was highlighted through one of Australia's 'wisdom writers', Anne Deveson. In her book *Resilience* (2003) she begat a language that sprang from her definition and exploration of where her own remarkable resilience came from, having experienced the suicide of a schizophrenic son and the death of her partner from oesophageal cancer.

What can be called 'the resilience movement' can be seen as based on her definition: 'Resilience is the life force that flows and connects every living thing, continually prompting regeneration and renewal' (p.267). Her statement identifying the basic need of all humans for 'connectedness' sent out a clear message to GPs about their proactive role in the community.

It was apparent that a jigsaw was coming together: in community understanding, in child psychology and practice, in bullying prevention in commerce and schools, suicide prevention, psychiatric research and in general practitioner training. The word 'resilience' is now in common use in Australia and the possibility of promoting it acknowledged as an important part of personality development.

In 2006 my article entitled 'Resilience promotion and its role in clinical medicine' was published in the *Australian Family Physician*, the journal of the Royal Australian College of General Practitioners (Lloyd 2006). This restated the important role of empathy in the GP–patient relationship. The use of phrases leading to basic feelings was promoted to indicate to the patient that their primary carer understands the darkness, isolation and loneliness of their struggles. This represented an anchor from which their ability to bounce back – their resilience – could start to be regenerated. This approach is the essence of making contact with those in the darkness of a dementia situation.

This represented a huge task for the time-pressed and partly burnt-out GP, particularly if the philosophy of supporting the whole person is not accepted as a responsibility. Fortunately, since 2007 the Australian health care system allows delegation for this type of support to psychologists. This was partly due to the depression epidemic that has been identified in our country, particularly among rural farmers affected by the climate change.

A presentation at a weekend for GPs generated a resilience promotion model that has been found very acceptable for self-assessment and in small groups (Figure 13.3). It avoids asking direct questions about religion but paces the discussion suitable to the particular dynamics of the group. Working with this model leads into surprising areas; ones not easily approached by many people.

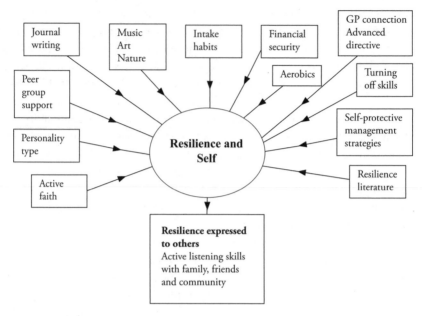

Figure 13.3 Resilience factors for GPs

Particular points should be noted in the model depicted in Figure 13.3:

- *Resilience for others*
  A resilient therapist or person is much more likely to be able to promote resilience in another person; self-care is an important professional need often neglected.

- *Personality type*
  Getting behind difficult behaviour can be enhanced if staff can learn that excessive demands and expectations from a patient can be part of a lifelong mindset generated by childhood neglect. This approach generates a more tolerant approach with a case management focus.

- *Turning off*
  The current older generation often lacks mind-control skills that are useful for dealing with insomnia and chronic pain or creating positive mental images that can deal with depression. Generating interest in practising them may be difficult but can be gently presented in a session in which music is a part.

- *Advance care directives*
  This neglected strategy – known to some as a 'living will' – provides a document in which a person gives instructions about his or her

future health care and asserts his or her rights as a patient (Graham *et al.* 2004). It comes into effect only when the person is no longer capable of making decisions.

TURN OF THE TIDE

In Australia the tide is turning; the resilience jigsaw is coming together rapidly. Other countries may be differently placed, but the height of awareness of the strategy of the resilience promotion model can be seen as an indicator of community resilience, and of the status of aged care residential culture.

But there is still a problem at university level. David Tacey of LaTrobe University in Melbourne, in his book *The Spirituality Revolution* (2003, p.201), wrote: 'Spirituality is not on the training agenda in medical school and health professionals frequently feel unprepared to engage the spiritual longings or aspirations of their clients.'

Currently in Australia, the tightly protected technical approach of medical syllabuses is clearly under great pressure from some general hospitals, the palliative care sector and the awareness being raised in GP training. The importance of looking inside for the spiritual/resilience support that is there to protect us, if we can touch base with it, is now coming into prominence.

My own experience strongly suggests that the necessary changes in the system will not come from the conservative bureaucracy of church or medical faculty but will flow gradually from the innovative hospitals, faculties and general practitioners. The culture and trend in the UK and elsewhere may well be different, but the power games are likely to be the same.

SINGING GROUPS AS RESILIENCE PROMOTERS

Using the firm footing provided by the resilience promotion approach, there are some administrative questions that should be asked under the troubled heading of 'cost rationing'.

- What is the most effective way to promote resilience in the elderly, especially those with dementia?

- Is there an approach which is non-threatening, compact and does not place further demands on a labour force that is always likely to be too small?

My work as a volunteer has shown that volunteer-supported singing groups are an avenue of opportunity that is cost-effective, non-threatening and practical. It lights up the often unrecognised residual brain function of the brain-damaged person and provides moments that are really heart-warming.

While visiting choirs represent great stimulus and entertainment, there is a high risk that choir visits will be infrequent and will use the choir's favourite and rehearsed numbers that do not facilitate the audience to join in. The audience is 'sung at' rather than 'sung with'.

The use of familiar music combined with the connectedness that can be achieved by identifying songs that have a special relevance to the person introduces members of the group to one another and also produces 'golden moments' for both co-ordinator and group. It takes advantage of the mystical ambience created when people sing, particularly when they find they can let fly without being told they are awful.

The background to the program that has been developed is expressed in the verse of the song 'As long as I have music' (Besig and Price 1986):

> For as long as I have music,
> As long as there's a song for me to sing,
> I can find my way; I can see a brighter day.
> The music in my life will set my spirit free.

This sets the theme that establishes the validity of using singing as a basic approach in residential villages.

In the UK, under the banner of 'Singing for the Brain' (Alzheimer's Society 2010) and with the backing of the Alzheimer's Society, there are already some 30 groups in the south and south-west of England. This sends out a challenging wake-up call to the Australian system, where the awareness of this approach is developing slowly, prodded by an interesting background.

In 2008/9 'The Choir of Hard Knocks' program on ABC TV provided a vivid demonstration to the community of how disadvantaged people can be given 'rehabilitation of the soul' – a return of self-esteem, drive and resilience – through the combination of singing and the teamwork and bonding that is achieved in a choir environment.

There is a very strong evidence base in the general and clinical literature that music is good for physical and emotional health. Two key books in this area give numerous and heart-warming examples of the impact of music on both normal and mentally disabled people.

The Mozart Effect by Campbell (1997, p.161) notes: 'Ambient music is not created to entertain or stimulate the intellect, but to act upon the body and emotions, helping us to reclaim our inner landscapes, restore spaciousness in our lives and reconnect with the inner rhythms of nature.' World renowned neurologist Oliver Sacks in his book *Musicophilia* (2007) reviews many cases from his clinical experience. In a chapter on dementia he points to the importance of music as a key therapy for an area where there is a rapidly growing need: 'Music is no luxury to those lost in dementia but a necessity, and can have a power beyond anything else to restore them to themselves, and to others, at least for a while' (p.347).

There is a well-documented problem of depression in older people's residential villages in Australia (Fleming 2001; Lloyd 2004). A recent paper published by Kirstin Robertson-Gillam (2008) has provided a clear-cut evidence base confirming that this area of need can be met productively:

> Participating in a choir can enable an elderly person to be creative through the sheer enjoyment of singing with others and discussing life's memories sparked by the song material. To do this in the company of like-minded people improves awareness and increases a sense of personhood. By being in the choir, feelings of excitement for something new and unexpected to happen were stimulated. Choir members became aware that they could create something new from within themselves. (Robertson-Gillam 2008, p.186)

In the far South coast town of Batemans Bay, New South Wales, the response to visits from a range of amateur choirs is invariably 'when can you come again?' The repertoires chosen are very likely to be rehearsed choir favourites that create a very welcome visit but do not specifically seek audience involvement. While, in theory, activity therapists may be able to explore and develop this territory, it also presents as one in which volunteers may become involved if they have the confidence to provide a regular session that offers a 'choir' component.

Trial and error in a pilot study was based initially on *The Ulverscroft Blue and Red Large Print Song Books* (1974, 1989), but other possibilities were sought and tried. The reminiscence factor was actively explored when appropriate, and songs from non-Australian sources were sought and utilised. Some examples define the personal affirmation technique used.

- 'The road to Gundagai', with its reminder of 'Dad and Dave', a radio show in the thirties, established itself as a firm favourite.

- An East Prussian-born man led us in 'Lilli Marlene' in English, but with a variation in one verse in its original German language.

- A Russian lady was affirmed by the discovery of the Cossack-based melody for 'Those were the days'.

- A withdrawn Italian lady got involved with 'Santa Lucia' and proceeded to teach us the correct pronunciations.

- Wartime hit 'The Lambeth walk' produced an activity component, using modified steps assisted by walking frames.

With great subtlety, if a member of staff passed by, 'Bless this house' was sung. The most popular song, used to close all sessions, was 'Let there be peace'.

The key of recorded music was invariably found to be too high and a pitch tuner was used to set the key. A repertoire of six numbers was prepared and used for 'Happy Hour' gatherings.

This project and the UK experience have validated the potential of an in-house 'choir' being coordinated by someone with some basic (but not expert) choir experience who is prepared to go with the flow as well as incorporating a reminiscence component. The choir component is a gentle one that does not expect good recall. Close partnership with the activities officer is essential.

It is planned to establish a song book and record kit that will be used to encourage individual members of the 130 Australia-wide singing groups in the 'Sing Australia' system (see www.singaustralia.com.au) to make a weekly visit to their residential villages.

The message here is that there is a job for volunteers to provide this type of golden moment as often as possible for the occupants of residential villages. This may stretch personal boundaries, but the rewards to a very deprived and isolated group of people needing as much resilience as they can generate are beyond any question.

CHAPTER 14

Sounding the Depths

A Reflection on the Challenge of Dementia to Religious Belief and Practice

Brian Allen

Out of the depths I cry to you, O Lord;
O, Lord, hear my voice.
Let your ears be attentive to my cry...

(Psalm 130: 1–2)

The staff of a nursing home noticed how a resident with a diagnosis of dementia walked up and down the corridors reciting something which to them (the staff) seemed religious. There was certainly a ritualistic feel to this pattern of behaviour as far as they were concerned. Could this be some profoundly prophetic utterance? The words 'out of the depths', repeated frequently, were recognisable as the opening lines of Psalm 130, as used in some funeral rites. When I met the resident she smiled at me as she removed the plastic slot-in clerical collar I was wearing at the time. She kissed it and returned it to me, saying, 'I don't think much to that.'

LEARNING TO RESPOND TO THE CHALLENGE

This encounter, amongst many others, has both challenged me and prompted me to listen as carefully as possible to the voice of people with diminishing mental powers, which articulates much of dementia's challenge to religious belief and practice in particular, and spiritual values in general. Responses to this challenge are relevant not only to the case of people with diminishing mental powers, of course; they have a much wider application.

Active listening to the person lies at the heart of person-centred care. This approach informed a two-day training course developed by two nursing home managers (Lesley Lee and Janice Paterson) and myself. This was designed for and delivered to care staff in our local mental health NHS

Trust. In theory, adopting person-centred approaches to caring for people with dementia seems relatively simple; in practice it is far from easy. Our main concern was to find effective ways of what might be involved in moving from what Kitwood (1997a) identified as the old culture of dementia care to the new culture. Between us we had considerable experience of dementia care mapping as developed by Kitwood and others at Bradford University, particularly in relation to medical research, and felt well versed in the principles of person-centred care upon which this tool is based.

The course started with an exploration of the different types of dementia, where the intention was not only to demonstrate the importance of diagnosis to access care and develop research, but also to highlight the limitations of a solely medical model of care and treatment (Allen 2008). Participants were able to recognise some of the ways in which different forms of dementia manifested themselves in the lives of people they looked after. They also became more aware of how someone may show signs of more than one form of diagnosable dementia at the same time. More important was the realisation that beyond the diagnosis each individual experiences dementia in their own way, according to many factors other than the physical or biological. Such factors include the psychological, social and spiritual dimensions of a person's life.

SHARING THE LIVED EXPERIENCE

The focus of most of the course material was on the lived experience of the person with dementia and the relationship between that person and others, particularly the careworker. The main challenge here was how to enter into that lived experience. In the case of many other diseases, even in the advanced stages, the subject will often be able to describe that experience to others. This is not necessarily so in the case of people with diminishing mental powers, particularly in the later stages of the disease, where interpretations of communication are much more complex and elusive.

TOWARDS EMPATHIC IMAGINATION

To be able to put oneself in another's shoes requires not only information gathered from others and by one's own careful observations, but also the employment of considerable imagination. Empathic imagination is an important component of person-centred care, as it is of both pastoral and practical theology. A simple role-play was used in the training, in which one participant assumed the role of 'Rosie', a person with dementia in need of some personal care. In pairs, care staff assumed the roles of workers adopting opposing approaches to responding to Rosie's needs, one task-orientated and the other person-centred. Afterwards the difference in outcomes was discussed, focusing on Rosie's experience of the two different approaches. The role-play demonstrated that a person-centred rather than a task-orientated approach was more effective in accomplishing a necessary care task; noticing the physical and emotional impact on Rosie was often a powerful prompt to empathic imagining, offering an insight into the lived experience of the person with dementia.

Empathy is often referred to as an essential element of good care in many contexts but it is also costly, especially in relation to people with dementia. Consideration of the emotional labour involved (Smith P. 1992) raises questions as to whether we can afford, in terms of the impact on carers, person-centred care (Gibson 1999). Barbara Pointon's (2007) moving description of her experience of caring for her husband Malcolm highlights the importance of paying attention to the person rather than the disease. She makes the point that this includes the person's spirituality, something which was essentially personal to Malcolm. This move from caring for the person with *dementia* to caring for the *person* with dementia (Stokes 2000) underpinned the training being described here.

SOME CREATIVE OPTIONS

The course introduced John Killick's recordings (Killick 2004) of how he listened to people with dementia in order to craft their words into poems to tell their stories, which he then read. Participants were asked to pay special attention to their emotional reaction to listening to these readings; responses included both laughter and tears. We also used an extract from Tony Nicholson's televised drama 'Black Daisies for a Bride' (Nicholson 1994) in which people with dementia on Whernside Ward at the former High Royds Hospital near Leeds were at the centre of the play as their stories were unfolded. At one point an entertainer arrives, gaudily dressed, accompanying himself on a banjo and performing the song 'You Beautiful Doll'. Course participants were asked once again to monitor their thoughts and feelings as they watched the video clip. Despite some mixed responses to the physical environment and the apparent intrusion of the visitor, what was most striking was the information that the residents' responses to this event revealed about their life stories: their hitherto hidden life stories and capacities became manifest.

The message emerges that all behaviour is meaningful communication requiring special attention which employs a careful and enquiring use of imagination. Creative media, including music, poetry, art and drama, assist in the search for this imaginative awareness of the depths of another person's lived experience. The Opera Group's production of *The Lion's Face* by Langer and Maxwell (2010), based upon the experience of dementia, is an excellent recent contribution to the repertoire of stimuli to this end.

ADOPTING A MINDFUL APPROACH

Paying attention, in the present moment, on purpose and non-judgementally, are basic elements of mindfulness approaches of caring for ourselves and others (Kabat-Zinn 1994). The intention to notice what is happening without criticism or analysis can lead to a greater awareness of how things are (Shapiro *et al.* 2006). Such awareness can create space within which it becomes possible to see things differently; we may not be able to change events, but we can sometimes change our relationship to them.

Mindful practice was employed in preparation for some guided visualisation where the course participants were invited to enter a scenario in a care setting and observe one individual's responses to activities in a short time-span. They were then asked to turn their attention to a series of questions about the meaning they might attach to what they had observed, and how this connected with individuals' life stories. This provided another opportunity to employ empathic imagination as a way to access the lived experience of the person with dementia.

ELLEN'S PRAYER

Adopting a compassionate mind (Gilbert 2009), one of the potential fruits of mindfulness practice, not least towards oneself, is a simple concept but requires persistent practice to be able to apply it to life's many complex situations. In this respect it is much like prayer in the sense that commitment is required to practise adopting an open and compassionate relationship between one's self and another. Sometimes this is quite explicitly so, as in the case of Ellen's prayer, portrayed in the Christian Council on Ageing's short film *Is Anyone There?* (Arthey 1997). This arose out of a dementia project based in Newcastle-upon-Tyne and was used in the training described here. Ellen was a life-long practising Roman Catholic with a past and future, but for whom meaning is to be found in present-moment encounters. During Ellen's final years in a nursing home the chaplain (Audrey Ball), a

Roman Catholic Eucharistic minister, used to walk in the grounds, as well as sit, talk and pray with her, before administering the sacrament of Holy Communion. The chaplain commented:

> One lady I've been visiting regularly now for over a year, and for quite a long time I was able to give her Holy Communion. And when she became more distressed and disturbed it wasn't always possible. But we always prayed. I would say, 'Shall we pray now?' and she would always say the same thing, 'That's the best'. But one day it was different and we went for our usual walk. When we came to sit down and I said, 'Shall we pray now?' before I could even start a prayer she had started one of her own:
>
>> Dear God
>> You are all that matters
>> Help us to be happy
>> Help us to be welcoming
>> We need each other.
>
> I've had to learn not to become frustrated and not to judge what might be going on between one person and another in prayer. Something very special to me is the sacrament of the present moment. A person with dementia lives in the present moment. (Arthey 1997)

THE SPIRITUAL DIMENSION AS ESSENTIAL TO PERSON-CENTRED TRAINING

Using this kind of material reinforced the importance of listening to the voice of the person with diminishing mental powers. The example above comes from the Christian tradition, but participants were encouraged to be aware of diverse religious traditions (Allen 2002) and how they might be expressed both verbally and non-verbally.

The training described above included exercises to identify what contributed to the participants' own wellbeing and ill-being; they realised that it was much the same for people with dementia. Different modes of communication were explored and an introduction to dementia care mapping was also provided. Within this context the inclusion of the spiritual dimension as essential to person-centred care was accepted and positively evaluated.

The experience of caring for people with diminishing mental powers and developing training to promote person-centred care in this way highlights some fundamental issues in relation to personhood, spirituality and dementia. What follows is a brief outline of some reflections on these issues.

WORDS AND MEANINGS, ACTIVITY AND PASSIVITY

To read someone 'as if they were an open book' supposes that meanings may be taken at face value. However, words show something beyond themselves; we need to reflect on more than just the printed page, as it were, to understand what is being said. Perhaps, if we regard persons as living documents, we need to read between the lines to reach their meanings and thereby develop what we might call an interlinear interpretation of, or approach to, understanding their personhood (Allen and Coleman 2006).

Ellen's prayer, for example, was offered by a person out of the depths of her experience of dementia. It could be interpreted as addressing the Other, the ground of our being, the 'I am that I am', about the importance of our shared moods and feelings and recognising our essential interdependence. Such an insight comes out of the depths of her experience of increasing diminishment and articulates something of the 'divinisation of [her] passivities' (Chardin 1960, p.49 ff). Although she had no control over what was happening to her, she gave voice to meaning in the midst of her situation. In his spiritual classic *Le Milieu Divin* (1960) Teilhard de Chardin finds meaning not only in the activities of life but also in its passivities. Here is a world view which accommodates human passivities, including death: 'Death is the sum and consummation of all our diminishments' (p.61). Chardin meditates on the divinisation of our passivities and sees death not so much as the ultimate moment at which we receive the sacrament of Holy Communion; he invites us to consider death itself as the ultimate act of Holy Communion.

SUFFERING AND THE UNCHANGING NATURE OF PERSONHOOD

The unchanging nature of the divine personhood is consistently compassionate. Out of the depths of human experience, meaning can be constructed and recreated. Viktor Frankl demonstrates the significance of finding meaning in the apparently least significant events as a means of people maintaining their humanity, as he observed during the Holocaust (Frankl 1984). The two World Wars of the twentieth century have focused much thinking, such as that of the former prisoner of war and theologian Jurgen Moltmann (1974) on the nature of suffering.

In Christian thought the focus has become more on God's involvement in suffering in the person of Christ, thereby challenging the concept of God's nature as unchanging. Another view submits that in the Christian tradition God is viewed simultaneously as unchanging and yet suffering, both attributes being essential to one another (Castelo 2009).

The Old Testament attributes both passion and transcendence to God. Talk about God's transcendence has to be complemented by talk of his promise to be intimately involved with humanity. 'The importance... of the confession "Jesus is Lord" is not only that Jesus is divine but that God is Christlike. God is Christlike and in him is no un-Christlikeness at all' (Ramsey 1969, p.98). Christ suffered indeed, but did so without his essential nature being changed. Therefore, to say that we are made 'in the image of God' implies that whilst we suffer, we yet remain fundamentally the same person.

Herein lies an apparent contradiction and the point at which it is necessary to acknowledge divine mystery or paradox. A popular portrayal of this ancient problem of the nature of God's relationship to suffering is to be found in *The Shack* (Young 2007), in which the relationship between the different persons of the Trinity, Father, Son and Holy Spirit, is an essential feature of the drama. Each needs the other as they enter the realm of suffering and yet they remain in essence themselves. This is an image or model of human interdependence in the face of suffering which challenges us to suffer with one another and yet remain ourselves.

WE NEED EACH OTHER

Ellen's prayer echoes John Donne's famous sermon in which he claims:

> No man is an island entire of itself; everyman is a piece of the Continent, a part of the main; if a clod be washed away by the sea, Europe is the less, as well as if a promontory were; any man's death diminishes me, because I am involved in Mankind; and therefore never send to know for whom the bell tolls, it tolls for thee. (Donne 1987, p.87)

Some would argue that it is a self-evident truth about human nature that no one exists in isolation. Nonetheless, the prevalence of individualism and the emphasis on individual identity and capacity can undermine this approach, both in theory and in practice.

Countering this Western individualism is the African notion of *Ubuntu*. The word originates from several of the languages of southern Africa and emphasises the interconnectedness and relatedness that is essential to both personhood and nationhood. Gooder (2009) suggests that this is innate, and tells of her own very young daughter who, when asked to draw a picture of herself, drew several figures in the one picture. When asked about this, the child's simple explanation was that this was a picture of her and her family; she could not separate her identity from those to whom she knew she belonged.

Listening to the lived experience of people with dementia and their carers inevitably poses some basic questions about ourselves. Existential questions about personal identity and destiny, meaning and purpose are fundamental to recent explorations of spirituality. Such explorations have often taken place in the past within the framework of faith as both the means and the end of the spiritual quest. Religious belief and practice is not without its critics, of course. History demonstrates the abuse of religion, which can be described as the politics of spirituality. Such political realities, as well as the development of philosophical thought, have often led to the belief that questions about who we are and what is to become of us can no longer be answered adequately in religious terms. The task in this context is to rediscover possible meanings of such key concepts as 'person' and 'individual' which may have become lost in modern and post-modern thinking. Indeed, they may not have been developed adequately to be sustainable, in theory or in practice.

BECOMING PERSONS

Is there a point at which it can be said that the person with diminishing mental powers is no longer a person? In the severe stages of the disease it is not uncommon for observers to comment that someone is no longer 'the person they used to be'. Clearly they have not become someone else – so have they become less than a person? It is helpful to think here of the 'unbecoming' self as still being the self, despite changes in behaviour and communication. Brennan comments on the philosophy of both Locke and Hume on this topic; his option is 'to note the more modest possibility that personhood itself may be a matter of degree' (Brennan 1990, p.158.). He considers that Locke's definition of a person as a being with reason and reflection that can 'consider itself, the same thinking thing, in different times and places' lays an unsuitably high expectation on what it is to be a unitary person. Similarly, Hume's view that a person is no more than the sum of their experiences would seem to be too limiting. There is a point at which it is not possible to talk about ourselves without reference to others.

The theory underpinning the new culture of dementia care (Kitwood1997a), referred to in the training outlined above, owes much to the Jewish writer Martin Buber (Buber 1958) and the way in which dialogical personalism has been interpreted in practice. Much is required of the carer to maintain a positive regard for someone with dementia as a person. Both are themselves in relation to the other. Faith Gibson (1999) has questioned the demands made upon carers by the high standards set by Buber's concept of dialogical living, as interpreted and applied by Kitwood and others. However, we can do nothing less, Gibson proposes, for to ignore one person's diminishment would be to diminish us all (cf. Donne). Whilst people with dementia require much from others, they can also show others much about the range of human communication, and therefore much of what it is to be human. Buber declares, 'The primary word I–Thou can only be spoken with the whole being' (Buber 1958, p.11). Thus, if we are to understand the human experience of dementia, it is essential to see personhood in relational terms.

PERSONS, NON-PERSONS AND CREATION

Spiritual and pastoral care of people with dementia (Allen 2010) can be said to be based upon an unconditional, person-centred approach in which (for example) the foundation for Christian ministry is centred on the personhood of Christ, who embodies suffering and undying love. However, much of the Western tradition shares a view of 'persons' defined by function and rationality, which makes dysfunction and irrationality indicative of non- or sub-persons. This implies comment on a society that is itself unable to cope when confronted by apparent weakness and dependence, seeing it as meaninglessness and failure.

Such attitudes, often born out of fear, can achieve the semblance of moral and political acceptability which makes it is possible to dispense with those whose brains malfunction, as in the case of thousands of mental hospital patients in Nazi Germany: the German psychiatrist Alfred Hoche used the word *Ballastexistenzen* (human ballast) to designate people whom society could dispose of without losing anything essential. This blasphemes the Creator, who connects them inseparably through that same creation to others with apparently well-functioning brains. Deviation and diminishment are natural parts of purposeful and loving divine creativity. The Creator is involved within the creation and shares risk and self-exposure to ambiguities and 'failures'. The creation communicates with the Creator with groans beyond words (Romans 8: 26), and even the elements worship their creator (the 'Benedicite').

RELATIONSHIP AND DIVERSE PERSPECTIVES

Martin Buber's classic *I and Thou* (1958) influences much of Kitwood's promotion of the new culture of dementia care, which sees people with dementia as primarily persons and persons in relationship. Buber describes life as dialogue: in the beginning is relationship. Buber argues that both the personal and communion between persons cannot be reduced; the place where meaning is found is within the communication of the one with the other/Other. Commenting on this, Robinson (1997, p.9) writes:

> In the beginning and in the end is relationship, which can never be transcended or absorbed – even in God. There is the closest possible mystical unity between I and Thou, but always it is a mysticism of love, which insists upon and respects the non-identity of the other.

John Robinson draws upon Buber in this discussion about the significance of dialogue, seeking to show how the apparent opposites contained within Christian and Hindu belief systems in fact belong together. Robinson makes the point that this argument could be pursued by an examination of yet other religious traditions and their relationships one to another.

This demonstrates the centrality of dialogue to the study of religions, and how such dialogue might enrich our understanding of the human lived experience and cast light on the present discussion. For example, in her hitherto unpublished research amongst literate populations of similar socio-economic backgrounds in Chennai and Newcastle-upon-Tyne, Elizabeth Mukaetova-Ladinska (Newcastle-upon-Tyne University) suggests that there could be some correlation between the low prevalence of dementia in the Indian sub-continent and religious belief and practice.

Within Christianity the Eastern tradition in particular regards the doctrine of the Trinity as the primary image of divine relationship, as exemplified in the renowned icon by Andrei Rublyov, an image which can help inform approaches to personhood and people with dementia, as described elsewhere (Allen and Coleman 2006).

MEMORY AND SOCIAL RESPONSIBILITY

Where memory is problematic, not least for guaranteeing continuity, being remembered by God in 'the land of forgetfulness' (Psalm 88:12) is an expression not only of faith, but also one which raises the question as to where memory may be located. Rather than limited by being defined as a function of the individual, memory is seen as something that resides in community, tradition and place, and so is not entirely dependent on any one individual's level of cognitive function. Clearly the practice of communities observing ritual and a special sense of place, or sacred space, as a way of 're-membering' is not the monopoly of any one tradition. Belonging to and being remembered by both church and society is a particularly significant theme in relation to people with dementia. Identity and meaning for people with dementia are preserved through the community that remembers and cares for them.

The Church of England's report *Ageing* (Board of Social Responsibility 1990) refers to Hugo Petzch's study (1984) of societal attitudes to people with dementia, where he describes three models. These are biblical models which arise out of reflecting upon times spent working among people suffering with dementia.

The 'scapegoat' model (Leviticus 16) reflects some of the least favourable attitudes, where the need to distance oneself from the victim and to avoid any fear of contamination by association are both present. Those who are put out of sight bear the burden of the guilt of society for the breakdown in relationships.

The image of the suffering servant provides the second model, where the servant's plight and the onlookers' responses (Isaiah 53: 2–4) show the collective nature of the problem. The restoration of broken relationships can begin when we recognise that our own attitudes play a part in distancing others, including people with dementia. The health service and churches may both operate in this way when they publish reports which all too often lead to 'informed inertia'. Care, similarly, may reflect such attitudes by focusing on practical and physical tasks alone; people with dementia may become valuable objects as potential brain tissue donors to assist medical research. Petzch argued that the first two models overlap, and that people often shift between them in the attitudes that they express.

Petzch's third model seeks to establish a more appropriate response to the problem of our relationship with people whose cognitive functioning is disturbed and diminishing. This draws upon the New Testament account of the Gadarene demoniac (Luke 8), where the emphasis is upon someone rejected by society being called by name, offered unconditional acceptance (i.e. not subjected to the 'malignant social psychology' of infantilisation, outpacing, objectification and so on), and the saving act culminating in the person's restoration to society. Here Petzch stresses that the will to restore the person is a prerequisite. Unconditional acceptance will bring concern for the plight of sufferers who are otherwise rejected, and the will and means to alleviate the suffering, even if at present it is incurable, can follow.

These models are, of course, provisional but are also representative of much of the recent history of care of people with dementia (especially severe dementia), and of experiences to which some carers, both relatives and professionals, bear witness. It could be argued that since the early 1990s there has been important progress in the cause of person-centred approaches to people with diminishing mental powers and their carers. Kitwood and others have done much to confront the 'malignant social psychology' which operates to the detriment of people with dementia to the degree that they are regarded as less than persons. Nonetheless, a radical pastoral and practical theology is needed in order to respond to the challenge dementia makes to religious belief and practice. Such a response will reinforce and deepen the call to ensure that people with diminishing powers and their carers are treated as full human beings, made in the image of a loving creator and entitled to be treated as citizens as much as anyone else. Out of the depths of human experience and suffering they call not only to God but to the whole of humanity, to whom they inextricably belong.

CHAPTER 15

'They Maintained the Fabric of this World'

Spirituality and the Non-Religious

Malcolm Goldsmith

INTRODUCTION

A few years ago I remember a friend talking to me about his father's funeral. There was a service in church, which he and his mother were very keen to have, but they struggled with the fact that his father never went to church. My friend reasoned that if he never went to church when he was alive, was it morally acceptable for them to take him there when he was dead? In the end they reached a compromise solution: they all went to the funeral in church, but when they got there they left the coffin outside, in the porch. Mother and son said their prayers and gave their thanks and then they rejoined his father as they left the church.

I often thought of this when I was called upon to conduct the funerals of men and women who had no connection whatsoever with the church. Sometimes I didn't know them and I would piece together an understanding of their life from my conversations with the relatives. Sometimes this took a long time, but it was important, since it was a way of recognising their individuality and honouring them in that process. But sometimes I did know the deceased people and very often knew them to be lovely, upright and generous, even though they might not have been particularly religious. It was always a challenge to provide a funeral service which didn't pretend that they were other than what they were, but which also allowed family and friends to pay their respects and to mark with integrity the passing of a life.

I was always helped in this process by reflecting on verses in Chapter 38 of the book Ecclesiasticus (1970) which is to be found in the Apocrypha, that collection of books in many (but not all) Bibles between the Old and New Testaments. The writer observes that 'a scholar's wisdom comes from ample leisure; if a man is to be wise he must be relieved of other tasks'. We might use slightly different words in today's world, and of course the demarcations within society are different now, but the thrust of the writer's argument is clear: that most people are too busy getting on with life to have the time or opportunity to engage with what he regarded as the higher things of life. He writes about the ploughman, 'who is absorbed in the task of driving oxen and talks only about cattle'. He writes about craftsmen and designers who 'sit up late to finish their task'. 'So it is with the smith, sitting by his anvil'…so it is with the potter, sitting at his work, who 'stays awake to clean out the furnace'. These men, the writer asserts, rely upon their hands and they are skilful at what they do. If they did not exist then cities would not be able to function and societies would collapse, because everyone relies upon them. Then come these wonderful words – *'but they maintain the fabric of this world, and their daily work is their prayer'.*

These, to me, are the vast majority of the non-religious people of our world. Good, honest, hard-working people who have brought up their families, faced good times and bad, won some battles and lost a few as well, who have done what has been necessary to earn their living and contribute to the life of their families, their communities and to society in general. Rich and poor, well educated and not so well educated, political and apolitical – they are a mixed lot and, together with other people who may have found some meaning and significance in religious faith and practice, they make up the world that we know.

Just as these people deserve funerals which honour and respect them, so, when they grow older and perhaps develop dementia and need some form of residential care, they deserve their core being to be recognised and nurtured in a way that honours and respects them without assumptions being made. Whatever it is that is at the heart of people, whatever it is that gives meaning and significance to their life, whatever it is that provides them with the will to continue, is at the heart of what, in recent years, has become known as spirituality. When my father-in-law, in his nineties, was admitted into a care home, my wife was sent a care plan and in the section headed 'Spirituality' there was a line drawn across the page with large letters 'N/A' (not applicable) written, because he was not a church attender! It is that sort of assumption that I wish to challenge.

PROBLEMS OF DEFINITION

We are immediately plunged into problems of definition. What is meant by spirituality? Is it acceptable to use a word that, for many people, has overtones of religion? Not necessarily because people are against religion, but rather because it suggests to them a whole area of life and experience that is not easily understood or embraced by them.

The term 'spiritual wellbeing' emerged after the White House Conference on Aging in 1971; it was a government initiative, of which the aim was to address spiritual wellbeing. After the conference many people tried to come to terms with what the term really meant (Harrington 2010b). An early attempt was made by Moberg (1979), when he suggested that it was:

> the wellness or 'health' of the totality of the inner resources of people, the ultimate concerns around which all other values are focused, the central philosophy of life that guides conduct and the meaning-giving centre of human life which influences all individual and social behaviour. (Moberg 1979, p.2)

Well, at least it was a start, and since then there have probably been several hundred attempts to define what exactly is meant by spiritual wellbeing or spirituality. There is a general acceptance now that it is a 'quality that goes beyond religious affiliation; that strives for inspiration, reverence, awe, meaning and purpose, even in those who do not believe in any god' (Goodall 2009, p.169).

Many people have tried hard to distinguish between spirituality and religion, suggesting that 'religious care is given in the context of shared beliefs, values and liturgies, whilst spiritual care is usually given in a one-to-one relationship' (Goodall 2009, p.169). That is a distinction I am not happy with, but at least it is an attempt to recognise some divide.

Another attempt came up with:

> spirituality is the quality of being concerned with deep feelings and beliefs (which are often religious) rather than with the physical parts of life. It is not solely confined to organised religion so someone can be spiritual without being religious. (Kemp and Wells 2009, p.333)

This was understood by Steindl-Rast and Lebell (2001), who wrote: 'sometimes people get the mistaken notion that spirituality is a separate department of life, the penthouse of existence. But rightly understood, it is a vital awareness that pervades all realms of our being' (quoted in Kemp and Wells 2009, p.334).

Perhaps we should listen more closely to what people with dementia themselves are saying. Christine Bryden writes:

The stigma of dementia leads to a view that we are beyond the reach of normal spiritual practices. But you can reach out to our true spiritual self that lies beyond cognition and emotion. You can help us to see beyond the transient worldly difficulties of coping each day with brain damage. Find out more about the unique individual who has dementia, about their preferences, and then find ways in which this person can be spiritually nourished. We can find meaning in our spirituality, and you can connect with us and empower us. (Bryden and MacKinlay 2008, pp.137–138)

Diana Friel McGowin approached the subject in this way:

my every molecule seems to scream out that I exist, and that this existence must be valued by someone! Without someone to walk this labyrinth by my side, without the touch of a fellow traveller who understands my need of self-worth, how can I endure the rest of this uncharted journey? (McGowin 1993, p.124)

We have yet to reach a satisfactory definition of spirituality which easily and openly includes both people with religious faith and those without, and which is not a latter-day revision of religious understanding to widen the gate a little so that others can be included. It is as though we now understand what we mean in terms of this approach to care and support for people with dementia, even though we have yet to find a word that is universally accepted to describe it. For the moment I am happy to go along with Mel Kimble's view that:

the spiritual dimension is the energy within that strives for meaning and purpose. It is the unifying and integrating dimension of being that includes the experience of transcendence…and the mystery that is at once overwhelming and fascinating, that renders my existence significant and meaningful in the here and now. It is also a mystery in that it is un-measurable, un-provable and lacks universal definition. (Kimble 2001, p.151)

At a much more mundane level, although vitally important, we are dealing with whatever it is that 'keeps a person's spirit up', and which does not make him or her 'dispirited' or 'low in spirit' or, as Froggatt and Moffitt (1997, p.225) put it, 'that which gives zest, energy, meaning and identity to a person's life in relation to other people and to the wider world'.

BEYOND DEFINITIONS

We are dealing with the area that Erikson (1982) grappled with, when people are living within a state of tension between integrity and despair. That struggle to maintain a sense of wholeness despite disintegrating physical or mental capabilities is of the essence of the search for a spirituality. It is that which affirms a person, no matter what his or her state, and gives a source of encouragement and hope and the means for possible growth and/or acceptance.

Koenig (1994, p.284) presents a list of 14 spiritual needs in ageing and it is interesting to note that only three of them have a specific religious reference. I place the latter at the end of the list, although that is not where he placed them. He writes about a need for meaning, purpose and hope; to transcend circumstances; for support in dealing with loss; for community; for personal dignity and a sense of worthiness; for unconditional love; to express anger and doubt; to love and serve others; to be thankful; to forgive and be forgiven; to prepare for death and dying; *for validation and support of religious behaviours; to engage in religious behaviours* and, finally, *to feel that God is on their side* (my italics). It can be said, of course, that all these needs are catered for in good and personalised care, and in many ways that is true, so why use the word 'spiritual' to describe them? However, in most care homes, how much time is left after the routine tasks of dressing and washing, eating and sleeping, exercise and recreation, to explore the inner depths of meaning, purpose and hope?

The response is usually that these routine tasks are not done in isolation but that they are, in themselves, the vehicles for enabling these other needs to be met. That, of course, is the hope and the intention, but in all honesty everyday practice falls far short of these ideals in the vast majority of care homes. 'The experience of living with dementia in residential care was fundamentally one of experiencing difficult and distressing emotions relating to loss, isolation, uncertainty, fear and a sense of worthlessness' was the conclusion reached by one team of researchers (Clare *et al.* 2008, p.711), and a report published by the Mental Welfare Commission for Scotland (2009, p.10) found that:

> some care homes had fallen seriously short of best practice and people with dementia were not always getting the best possible care to meet their needs...only 24 per cent of people had an adequate record of their life history...the quality of care reviews varied – there was rarely involvement of the person, with most reviews being carried out by care home staff and a relative or friend...around half of all the people never

went out of the care home and there was little planned activity outside the care home.

I am concerned that if many staff are unable to attend to these obvious needs, then how prepared and trained are they to deal with the more intangible areas of care, such as preparing for death and addressing issues such as a loss of meaning or a sense of despair? This is not meant to be a generalised criticism of care home staff, many of whom do superb work in situations of considerable difficulty where depression and dementia are the prevailing conditions (Dening and Milne 2009, p.40), but it is to recognise that we have a long, long way to go before we can be satisfied that residents receive the care that is needed if their inner (as well as their outer) needs are to be acknowledged and met.

THE UNIVERSALITY OF SPIRITUALITY

It is these needs and the ways in which they are addressed that form the basis of what we loosely call spirituality. People from a religious background will have the stories and practices of their faith to illuminate and describe many of these issues, but it is the issues that are central, and not the language we use to handle them. The question needs to be raised as to what language or images are available to people to address these issues if traditional religious language is no longer appropriate or relevant? It is my conviction that both religious and non-religious people need these issues and experiences to be explored and developed; they are the same issues whether a person is a religious believer or not. They will be handled in different ways by different people and it is not for any outsider to determine how, and by what means, individuals choose to address them. There is not one form of spirituality for the religious and another for the non-religious; there is a universal need to face up to issues of ultimate meaning and purpose, to recognise what gives vitality and hope to life in straitened circumstances, and to find ways to live at peace with the world, the neighbour and the self.

Joan Chittister (2003, p.61) puts it this way: 'Vulnerability renders all of us human, welcomes us into the human race, makes humanity an unbreakable bond…vulnerability is the call to self-acceptance, it is the great, liberating moment in the human journey.' Because people are different, by personality and by temperament, by upbringing and by experience, and by the situation in which they find themselves physically, mentally and geographically, they will journey in different directions. The important thing is that they move towards a sense of wholeness and peace, towards an acceptance of who they are now, rather than regret what they have been in the past.

NECESSARY COMPONENTS

So how can we help to establish an approach, a milieu, in which this can take place? Tom Kitwood (1997a, p.82) used a flower as an analogy, at the heart of which is love. Around that central part of the flower are the petals, and he describes five petals of comfort, attachment, inclusion, occupation and identity.

So, within a context of love – of compassion, acceptance, forbearance and understanding – a person needs to know the reassurance of comfort the derivation of which is COM-, Latin *fortis* 'strong' (*The Concise Oxford Dictionary*), that is, that the environment in which he or she lives is reliable and dependable, providing an undergirding of support and strength. The person needs to be able to form attachments, relationships with people, which means that despite possible, even probable, difficulties, he or she needs to be able to communicate, and those providing care need sufficient skill to be able to stay with the person until they are able to understand what it is that he or she is trying to communicate.

To give up on communication is to deny the person opportunities for meaningful or even possible relationships. When people's attempts to communicate are either ignored or misunderstood, then the likelihood is that they experience a form of rejection and protect themselves further by becoming more and more isolated, cutting themselves off from the very relationships which are necessary to sustain their dignity and their quality of life. To be excluded from the life of a community or from the possibility of friendship or reciprocal love is to be denied the metaphorical oxygen that is needed for living.

To be involved in some occupation which is significant is to have meaning, and where there is meaning to life there is hope and satisfaction, and yes, it is possible to have both, even in the midst of dementia. A sense of meaning is of the utmost importance, for without meaning there is little to prevent a decline into despair. Kimble and Ellor (2000, p.14) write that 'the vitality of a person's life, at every stage, depends upon his or her supply of meanings'.

When people lose the ability to tell or reflect on the story of their lives, they become dependent upon others to become the custodians of that story and therefore, ultimately, of that life. 'For those who have no living significant other, the *self* is all the more vulnerable' (Hepworth 2000, p.34). It is therefore vitally important that there are people around who can hold and keep alive those stories so that the person with dementia can maintain an identity, even though he or she may forget that identity. To the question

'Who am I?' we must answer: 'I am the stories and memories that I have about myself, plus the stories and memories that you have about me, plus the stories and memories that others have about me'. For the person with dementia the answer becomes 'I am the stories and memories that I *may* hold for myself, plus the stories and memories that you and others hold *for* me.' These are the components which, together, enable the person with dementia to remain a person, with an identity, a purpose and a community.

Fundamental to any understanding of spirituality is this commitment to honour a person's identity, to find meaning for his or her life, to encourage the possibility of relationship and to sustain a compassionate and secure environment in which the person can feel safe and also accepted. On paper these can seem simple requirements but in fact they are extremely difficult to recognise, establish and maintain. These are the fundamental needs of people, whether or not they are religious, and a commitment to them forms the basis of exploring and providing that climate of care which encompasses and embraces what is often called 'spiritual wellbeing'. It is an approach which has a profound effect upon both the receiver and the giver of care.

I was struck recently by the conclusions reached by a study of nurses engaged in long-term care in Canada (Parry 2009). After discussing the nature of compassion, seeing it as 'sensing another person's suffering combined with a desire to alleviate or reduce such suffering', Parry argues that all discussion about compassion which is not matched by an appropriate description of practical compassionate action is 'empty and meaningless'. She concludes:

> the individual is seen by the nurse as a whole person who does not just need to be washed, fed and changed, but a person who *deserves* to be washed, fed and changed – in a respectful, gentle manner that acknowledges the other's unique humanity. *Only a nurse who feels and conveys compassion can perform the essential ordinary tasks in this manner.* (Parry 2009, p.19) (my italics)

I believe that we can substitute the word 'carer' for the word 'nurse'.

This theme was explored more fully in one of the most thoughtful articles I have read in many years (McLean 2007). She claims that whenever care, concerned with body maintenance, is given without regard to the *person*, then an act of violence occurs. This exercise of strength over defenceless, failing and vulnerable bodies and spirits 'raises the spectre of immorality' (p.365). The article lifts the understanding of care-giving from being goal-directed tasks to being *relational transactions*. McLean argues that although care is a purchasable commodity, in an industry where caregivers themselves can be seen as purchasable commodities, the very nature of care and caregiving distinguishes it from other products. Care is essentially and necessarily inter-subjective, it is 'opening the self to another's inner life', it is a mutual relationship involving both caregiver and care-receiver, and when this relational dimension is missing, it is wrong to call the transaction 'care'. Bodies are attached to individuals, she argues, but persons are *produced* by human relationships, and in dementia, where there is so much fragility and vulnerability, 'they must be replenished continually'. The whole thrust of the article is to insist that authentic care is a process which changes both the giver and the receiver and, more than that, by its very nature, is a healing process.

All this, of course, is a development of the work of Martin Buber (1958), who distinguished between I–It relationships, where the person is regarded as an object (recalling Kitwood's (1997a) 'objectification' as one of the examples of a malignant social psychology) and I–Thou relationships, in which both participants are changed and grow by the mutual encounter. It is a meeting of equals, in which there is mutual respect, even though, as in dementia care, one party may be frail and vulnerable. In such a meeting, there is extra care needed on the part of the caregiver to ensure that there can be equality and not domination of one by the other. The discovery (and experience) of that equality is, in itself, of profound significance.

A moving example is described by Sally Knocker (2010) who tells how, when drawing the curtains one evening in a care home, she was struck by the sunset, so she turned to one of the residents and asked him if he would like to watch it with her:

> It is rare for me to enjoy total silence, but for 15 minutes we sat together without words enjoying this gentle spectacle in mutual awe and reverence. It was one of those unexpected experiences rarely to be shared or savoured so intimately with another person. (Knocker 2010, p.80)

They sat quietly together for a few more minutes before the resident, a man with dementia, turned to her and said in a whisper, 'That's what life is all about, isn't it?'

This can also be a demanding approach; it does not always, or perhaps often, come easily or quickly, but when it happens there is no mistaking its quality. Rosemary Clarke (2010) describes such an experience:

> I took comfort in being able to be with my mother in these ways. Together, I believe we were floating on a sea of unknowing, of

completely trusting. Sometimes I wept quietly, tears of loss, but also of letting go. I felt very relaxed, even serene and at peace in myself. The imminence of her passing was not a worry, but the herald, I somehow knew, of a moving on for her…and for me, to a different kind of rest. And I too surrendered now to 'whatever is'. I had arrived at what is perhaps called by religious people a state of grace. (Clarke 2010, p.207)

CONCLUSION

When I visit a care home and see 10 or 20 people sitting in a room or walking up and down the corridors, what do I see? Certainly I see frail, vulnerable and elderly men and women, but I also see people who have endured a great deal, who have created much, who have loved and been loved. People whose lives have created the society in which I live, and for which I am grateful. These are the people who have maintained the fabric of this world, and perhaps for most of them, their daily work has been their prayer. And what do I wish for these men and women? My wish is that they can live their final days with a sense of dignity and honour, that they can find some form of meaningful relationship with others and with their own inner being. My wish is that they may discover and maintain an inner peace and a sense of wonder, and that those who care for them engage with them in such a way that lives are transformed, and that even the simplest and most mundane task can be, using religious language, 'sacramental', although they do not need the religious language. Spirituality is as relevant for the non-religious as it is for the religious, because it is about the fundamental meaning of being human.

CHAPTER 16

Being in the Moment

Developing a Contemplative Approach to Spiritual Care with People who have Dementia

John Swinton

Dementia is amongst the most challenging mental health problems faced by society today. The life experiences of people with dementia offer profound challenges to the values, expectations, hopes and presumptions which form the very heart of the value systems of modern liberal Western culture.

Dementia scares us because it seems to take away all of the features that we have been taught are central to what it means to be human: the ability to 'have a voice', to articulate one's ideas in a meaningful fashion, to be a 'self-advocate', to have the capacity to assert one's position apart from any necessary relationship with or dependence on others. In a social context within which 'clarity of mind and economic productivity determine the value of a human life' (Post 1995, p.3), people with dementia stand awkwardly on the borders of acceptable humanness. In a 'hypercognitive society' (Post 1995, p.17) within which quality of life is judged in accordance with such criteria as usefulness, independence, rationality, productivity, vitality and fitness, one is constantly faced with the question: in what sense can those who appear to have been stripped of such things be viewed as living worthwhile lives? For some, the loss of memory and cognitive decline which mark dementia inevitably move sufferers out of the world of persons and into a strange land of 'invalidity', where, in significant ways, their personhood is deemed in-valid.

But if we probe a little deeper, we quickly discover that many of the 'common sense' assumptions that surround the experience of dementia are not quite as clear or as sensible as they appear. Take, for example, the presumption that dementia is a neurological condition. 'Surely,' one might say, 'at least that is a given!' But is it? Think of it this way: how exactly do we come to know when a person has dementia? A person becomes forgetful, begins to lose a sense of who they are, who others are, and how they relate to the environment around them. We then describe this experience as dementia, assume it to be a neurological condition and act accordingly. Thus far that seems pretty straightforward.

However, Tom Kitwood (1997b) makes the point that whilst dementia may well relate to neurological damage, the actual causation of that damage may be significantly more complicated than we often think. In order to understand Kitwood's point we need to think carefully about the nervous system and how it actually functions, grows and develops. Unlike other organs, the brain and the nervous system are plastic. By this I mean that their shape, form and development are responsive to the environment and the experiences that a person has. As we encounter the world, as we engage in tactile and experience-generating activities, so the brain shapes and forms itself according to its interpretation of these experiences. Unlike toenails or hair, which just grow according to a predetermined genetic pattern, from birth a person's brain is shaped and formed by their experiences. Thus, for every external experience a person has, there is an internal correlate within the neurons and synapses of the brain. What happens in the world around us, our experiences, relationships, feelings and so forth, are all registered in and impact upon the developing neurology of our brain.

This connection between experience and neurological change is important for Kitwood in relation to dementia. While most would agree that dementia has neurological origins, he is not content to describe dementia purely or even primarily in terms of biological decline. Once we have interpreted the behaviour of a person who we then decide has dementia, we then give them the label: dementia sufferer, Alzheimer's victim, etc. Once ascribed, these labels have a profound impact on the way in which society responds to the individual who bears the label.

Dementia, for the reasons mentioned previously, has particularly negative connotations within Western societies. These negative connotations easily translate into negative relationships, isolation and poor approaches to care. Kitwood hypothesises that these negative social experiences may actually contribute to the process of brain degeneration. If that is so, the impact of negative perceptions and relationships with people with dementia is not only a social and relational problem for them, it may also contribute to neurological decline.

This point needs some clarification. Kitwood describes dementia in terms of 'malignant social psychology' (1997a, 1997b; Baldwin and

Capstick 2007). Malignant social psychology refers to social environments in which the forms of interpersonal interactions and communications that take place diminish the personhood of those people experiencing that environment. In describing dementia in this way, Kitwood challenges descriptions which give priority to neurological dysfunction as being prior to and wholly responsible for the symptoms of dementia.

Malignant interactions need not be perpetrated from intent or malice. Often they are brought about through thoughtlessness, lack of insight or a lack of awareness as to the negative effects of particular attitudes, actions, behaviours and relationships. Such malignant interactions produce negative self-esteem and diminish the personhood of people with dementia. If the model of brain-to-world interaction described previously is correct, such negative interactions may actually have neurological correlates. In other words, dementia may well have a neurological root, but the neurological damage that is caused by the pathology may be increased by negative interactions (or lack of interaction) with others.

We might think of the process of dementing in dialectical terms. The experience of dementia is not simply created by dysfunctional neurology, but rather it is brought about through the complicated dialectical interaction between neurological impairment and interpersonal processes (Adams 1996). Dementia is thus seen partly as the result of the ways in which society treats particular people. Dementia may be socially constructed, not only in the sense that it is a diagnostic category arising out of social interaction and discourse by the medical profession, but also in that it is the result of society acting upon individuals (Adams 1996). Dementia is as much *a relational disability* as it is a physical or neurological one.

This is an important observation. If dementia is a relational disorder, then perhaps relationships are the primary way that we should respond to people going through it? There is some evidence that, given the correct relational environment, a process of 'rementing' may be initiated wherein people can reclaim some of the faculties that appear to have been lost to the illness (Sixsmith, Stilwell and Copeland 1993). This is not to suggest that dementia can be cured through relationships. Rather it draws attention to the vital fact that the essence of what it is to be a person and to remain a person may lie not in neurology but in relationships. It may be in the realm of the relational that genuine care, growth and re-personalisation can be worked out, even in the midst of profound neurological decline. This suggestion sits in a strange tension with the standard scientific account of inevitable loss and decline.

THE PERSON IS LOST TO THE ILLNESS?

In the same way as the common-sense understanding of dementia as a neurological problem can be probed and challenged, so also we can probe and challenge other 'common-sense' assumptions, such as the suggestion that the person is lost to the illness. Laying aside for the moment the vexed question of what a 'person' is, we might ask precisely why people feel that the person has gone when they have dementia. Obviously there is the profound and tragic experience of forgetting and being forgotten and all of the experiences that emerge from this. Many of the things that are familiar to us in the individual are, or appear to be, no longer available and it is difficult sometimes to hold onto the fact that they might still be the same person they used to be. But does this mean they have been lost to the illness? Does this really mean that they have somehow 'lost their minds'?

As one reflects on the literature that surrounds dementia, one is struck by some of the language used, in particular the language that suggests that a person with dementia is somehow 'losing their mind', the assumption being that the profound forgetfulness of dementia is somehow equated with a loss of mind. Once the 'mind' has gone the person no longer exists. Dementia is assumed to somehow 'de-soul' the person, as Oliver Sacks puts it (Sacks 1985, p.28). Such thinking is of course deeply tied in with the type of cultural assumptions highlighted previously and the implicit and explicit Cartesian presumption that the mind is the seat of the intellect and the essence of what it means to be truly human.

We cannot here get into the complex philosophical issues that surround whether or not a person has a mind, or indeed precisely what a mind is. What we can do, however, is ask a naive question: how do we know anyone has a mind in the first place, never mind whether or not they have lost it? Think of it this way: in order for any of us to make sense of the world it is necessary for us to enter into a process of mind-reading. As we engage in any form of communication, I need to pick up on the clues you give to me, your body language, facial expression, the language you use, etc., and it is as I strive to process this mass of communication that I can begin to make sense of our encounter and understand, or at least speculate, as to what is going on in your mind. Within that process I inevitably bring my own assumptions, prejudices and ways of seeing the world, based on what I have been taught throughout my life. But even at the best of times I can only guess what is *really* going on in your mind. Indeed I can only speculate and assume that you have a mind!

Why, then, bearing in mind that most of the 'minding' that we do is guesswork, do we so easily (and willingly?) ascribe a lack of mind to people with dementia? Could this be an example of malignant social psychology? One of the participants in Jaber Gubrium's fascinating study of the way in which we construct our minds in community (1986) makes this point well. Talking about her husband who has advanced Alzheimer's disease, she says:

> How do you really know [his mind has gone], you don't *really* know for sure, do you? You don't really know if those little plaques and tangles are in there, do you?...how do I know that the poor man isn't hidden somewhere, behind all that confusion, trying to reach out and say, 'I love you, Sara'? [she weeps]

She has retained her *faith* that her husband is worth the benefit of the doubt; she retains her *hope* that there might be something more than people assume; she holds onto her *love*, a love that refuses to forget her husband even in the midst of his own forgetfulness. The mind is a communal entity. Holding onto the mind of a person with dementia is a communal process that requires faith, hope and love.

TELLING NEW STORIES

As a way of beginning to illustrate the points made thus far, I will turn to a story told by Oliver Sacks (1985) in his book *The Man who Mistook his Wife for a Hat*. Reflection on this story will open up the conversation in a helpful way.

Jimmy's story

Oliver Sacks is a neurologist who has written extensively on his experiences with people who have neurological conditions that are odd, sometimes disturbing and always deeply illuminating. It is important to keep in mind the fact that Sacks is a scientist and a neurologist, that is, that he and his world view have been formed in quite particular ways. Sacks relates the story of a man, Jimmy, a former sailor, whose memory had been destroyed by Korsakov's syndrome. Korsakov's syndrome is a specific form of dementia which is the product of long-term alcohol abuse. It leads to irreversible degeneration of the brain. One of its central features is profound memory loss. The loss is so profound that sufferers become people without a past or a future, interminably trapped in an eternal present and bound permanently within one period of time. People with this form of mental health problem are in a very real sense lost and unable to establish roots. Strangely, Jimmy could remember things prior to 1945…but nothing since then.

Sacks was deeply challenged by his encounter with Jimmy. He recalls spending time talking with Jimmy at length about his life and his memories prior to 1945. They had been talking for 20 minutes or so when Jimmy turned and looked out of the window. When he turned back he seemed surprised to see Sacks. In the space of seconds his conversation with Sacks had disappeared from memory and he was starting his encounter again as if the past had never happened. Sacks, a secular Jew with no apparent spiritual commitments, described Jimmy as 'de-souled'. The disease had stripped him of something essential to what he was as a human being. From the perspective of his neurological gaze Sacks felt that the person Jimmy had been had gone; something essential to him being a person at all was no longer present. His soul had gone.

However, while Sacks conceived of Jimmy as being in a sense absent from mainstream humanity and merely a shadow of the person he used to be, those close to Jimmy saw something different. Their faith in Jimmy was stronger and their narrative was hopeful. One of the nurses said to Sacks: 'Watch Jimmy in chapel and judge for yourself.' Sacks comments:

> I did, and I was moved, profoundly moved and impressed, because I saw here an intensity and steadfastness of attention and concentration that I had never seen before in him or conceived him capable of… Fully, intensely, quietly, in the quietude of absolute concentration and attention, he entered and partook of the Holy Communion. He was wholly held, absorbed, by a feeling. There was no forgetting, no Korsakov's then, nor did it seem possible or imaginable that there should be – clearly Jimmy found himself, found continuity and reality, in the absoluteness of spiritual attention and act. (Sacks 1985, pp.36–37)

From Sack's position as a neurologist, Jimmy's was a narrative of pathology, lost personhood, a broken soul and presumed hopelessness. His damaged neurology was assumed to determine the nature and quality of his life. Yet, when the faith, hope and love of the nurses 'forced' Sacks to listen to a different story; when he was asked to *get closer and watch carefully*, his perspective was transformed. His revised understanding resurrected the person (Swinton 2000) behind the label of Jimmy's condition and opened up new possibilities for care and understanding that reached beyond the boundaries of the biomedical model and into the mystery which is human life.

From Jimmy's perspective, his spiritual encounter allowed him to enter into a familiar narrative that provided him with an anchor and a sense of self that was otherwise missing from his life. The fact that he would have forgotten it almost immediately afterwards is a by the way. The intensity and power of that unique and special moment was the transformative force that made his life hopeful.

THE DANGER OF TRANSLATION

Many people who have been with people experiencing dementia will be able to identify with Jimmy's story. Time and again one is struck by the impact that worship can have on people with dementia. People who appear to be totally unresponsive for the vast majority of their time can suddenly spring into life when they hear the Lord's Prayer, or particular hymns or Bible readings. When one witnesses such intense spiritual moments, one becomes deeply aware that there is 'something more' to people with dementia and that there are hidden depths which are not plumbed by current assumptions and modes of care. Now, of course one might simply wish to reduce experiences such as these to residual memory, the last cognitive vestiges of the person that once was, and suppose that while they might *appear* to be there in times of lucidity, in *reality* they have been destroyed by the dementing process. However, unless we are totally convinced by the neurological description of dementia; unless we have been persuaded that the person really has been destroyed by the illness; unless we believe that people are really nothing more than the sum of their memories, why would we choose to frame the experience as nothing more than residual memories, other than because we have been taught to do so? Could it not be that dementia in a sense 'locks people in', in a way that makes them unreachable using current assumptions and methods? Could it be that enabling people to function within the spiritual dimension is in fact a *key* which can unlock the person and reveal dimensions of personhood that appear lost until they are encountered in the stillness of that spiritual moment?

Jimmy's story reminds us that it is not possible to gauge what level of comprehension a person with dementia is *actually* functioning at. Whilst outer appearances may well reflect chaos, forgetfulness and loss, there may well be hidden depths to the person that, if the key can only be found, may reveal new and healing perspectives on the situation. We need to learn to give people the benefit of the doubt.

In Jimmy's case, spirituality offered just such a key to the inner depths of his experience. It was in the intensity of the spiritual moment that Jimmy revealed to the world there was more to him than failing neurology. It is not possible here to argue about the ontological significance of Jimmy's particular faith position – that is, whether something external to his neurology was actually happening. It is, however, vital to note the *functional* significance of his spirituality for revealing something of the invisible inner workings of his soul.

LEARNING TO BE IN THE MOMENT

How, then, in the light of the discussions presented thus far, might we go about developing an understanding and a practice of spiritual care with people with dementia? In what follows I will focus primarily on people with severe dementia, that is, those whom many assume to have 'gone', but to whom we might still be willing to give the benefit of the doubt. However, as we will see, the perspective I lay out is applicable in all contexts.

I was recently listening to a lecture on biblical hermeneutics given by Professor John Goldingay, a professor of Old Testament at Fuller Seminary in the USA. At the beginning of the lecture he gave an invitation to his students to join him and his wife for a meal the following week. His wife, who has now sadly passed away, had severe multiple sclerosis at the time of the lecture. He informed the students that his wife probably wouldn't remember them or be able to communicate, but he urged them nonetheless to speak with her. He said, 'She probably won't remember you afterwards, but in that moment she will appreciate you.' Hearing that was an epiphany. The place of meeting is in the sacred, often fleeting moment of connection between the person with dementia and those who desire to relate to her.

Goldingay's brief comment straightaway took my attention to the Christian contemplative tradition. The contemplatives, through dedication and spiritual exercises, seek ways of moving beyond the intellect and towards a state where they are totally immersed in the love of God. In this immersion, time disappears and each moment merges into an ongoing experience of love. Unbounded by the confines of rationality and reason, the contemplatives strive to get to the place where they can experience God's love and learn to love God, not for what God might do, will do or can do, but simply for God's sake. Learning to love God simply for God's sake echoes precisely the ways in which God loves us, not for what we have or do not have, can or cannot do, but simply because we are. Goldingay's urging his students to enjoy the sacrament of the present moment with his wife takes us deep into a tradition of contemplative presence wherein the present moment becomes all that there is and God's enduring attention in the present moment becomes a primary and ongoing locus for revelation and worship. Jean Pierre de Caussade (1996, p.1) outlines something of this perspective thus:

> God still speaks today as he spoke to our forefathers in days gone by, before there were either spiritual directors or methods of direction. The spiritual life was then a matter of immediate communication with God... All they knew was that each moment brought its appointed task, faithfully to be accomplished. This was enough for the spiritually minded of those days. All their attention was focused on the present, minute by minute; like the hand of a clock that marks the minutes of each hour covering the distance along which it has to travel. Constantly prompted by divine impulsion, they found themselves imperceptibly turned towards the next task that God had ready for them at each hour of the day.

If we follow the insights of this tradition, perhaps the primary task of spiritual care with people who have severe dementia is to learn a new meaning for time and discover the deep spiritual significance of the present moment.

RE-THINKING TIME

In order to learn how to be with people in the moment, we need to begin by re-thinking our understandings of time. Jean Vanier is helpful on this point:

> Individual growth towards love and wisdom is slow. A community's growth is even slower. Members of a community have to be friends of time. They have to learn that many things will resolve themselves if they are given enough time. (Vanier 1989, p.80)

The idea of becoming friends of time is important for dementia care. One of the interesting things to note about capitalist societies is the way in which time has become a commodity. We 'buy time', 'sell time', 'waste time', etc. We live with time as if it is constantly about to run out! Time is often a deep source of frustration and angst. Rather than being friends of time, very often time becomes our enemy! But Vanier asks us to slow down and, as Stanley Hauerwas (1988) puts it, 'take time for the trivial'. We need to learn to live differently with time. Living differently requires that we recognise where it is that we are living. If 'the world' is actually creation, then we live in God's time. Living in God's time means, if nothing else, that time is deeply meaningful and purposeful.

Hans Reinders (2007, p.177) has noted that 'western culture is dominated by a secular notion of time, which entails that time has no meaning other than the meaning it acquires through human plans and purposes'. If we work with concepts of what Reinders describes as 'empty time', dementia will inevitably appear meaningless and purposeless. However, if we take seriously the notion of providential time, an idea that suggests that God has redeemed time and that we now inhabit an eschatological space that has a timeline that is radically different from the timeline of the world, then things begin to look different. Time is not empty (Kennison 1990). Each moment is filled with meaning and new possibilities and eschatological significance. If time is meaningful, then taking time to be with a person with severe dementia is meaningful and purposeful.

BEING IN THE MOMENT

Thus when we engage with a person with severe dementia, as we learn to be in the present moment with them and as we recognise the poignancy of that moment, so new life and fresh possibilities are injected. Our time is used well, even if the recognition of that moment is brief and passing. Spiritual care begins when we learn what it means to be 'in the moment' with people whose moments are fragmented and fleeting but nonetheless deeply meaningful.

I recognise that not every reader of this book will identify with the theological framework offered here. Nonetheless, the principle remains the same. Spiritual care with people who have severe dementia begins when we learn to recognise and value the significance of the present moment, and to utilise that knowledge to enable ourselves and others to see beyond the 'obvious'. When we do that we open up a space for relating within which the spiritual, in all of its diverse forms, becomes a conduit for 'being with' people with severe dementia in ways which are meaningful and transformative for all of us.

CONCLUSION

I began this chapter by stating that dementia is amongst the most challenging of mental health problems faced by society today. This is true. However, as we have moved through the various conversations in this chapter, it has become clear that the challenge is not necessarily as straightforward and obvious as we might at first assume. The challenge dementia offers is of course personal and tragic. My intention in this chapter has not been to try to downplay the suffering that dementia causes to individuals or their families. That remains very real. Nevertheless, there are challenges to established ways of thinking about and responding to dementia that offer new possibilities for hope and transformation even in the midst of the sadness and brokenness that accompanies the condition. My suggestion of returning to the spiritual insights of the contemplative tradition is but one way that we can re-think and reframe our responses to people with severe dementia. If we can learn to recognise each moment as a sacrament, then not only will we discover ways of being with people who have severe dementia, we will also discover new ways of being with and loving *all* people. If dementia brings any blessing at all, perhaps that is it?

CHAPTER 17

Personhood, Personalism and Dementia

A Journey of Becoming

Clive Baldwin

INTRODUCTION

It is my contention that much of what passes for 'person-centred care' is not only a pale shadow of what authors such Kitwood envisaged when suggesting that 'the person comes first' (Kitwood 1997a) but also philosophically and ethically confused. This might strike you, the reader, as an extravagant and unfair claim, given the remarkable improvements in dementia care since Kitwood's challenge of the standard paradigm, but I would ask you to set aside your initial misgivings and allow my argument a fair hearing.

My argument here is relatively straightforward – although appreciating the detail within the argument will require some effort – and is sequentially as follows:

- that implicit within much of current person-centred care is an essentialist conception of personhood rather than a dialogical or relational one

- that this essentialist view of personhood leads to the person living with dementia becoming the object of care and as such being managed (albeit caringly) within the system-world of dementia care.

In this system-world ethics is reduced to a subset of decision-making theory (that is, what is best for the object of care) rather than based on a relationship founded on situated encounters of embodied agents.

This relational view of ethics – drawn from authors such as Buber (1958) and Levinas (1961) – calls for criteria for ethical reasoning different from those presented by the dominant ethical framework of principlism.

These criteria can be found in an approach called personalism – though this itself requires further development and elaboration if it is to do full justice to the nature and demands of ethical encounters.

In outlining my argument I am aware that I am, and shall be, using a number of terms that might be unfamiliar: essentialist conception of personhood, principlism, system world, lifeworld, the Face, personalism, lines of flight, and so on. Rather than overwhelm with definitions at the outset, again I beg indulgence to allow me to explain these as I go along. I can only suggest that you return to the summarised argument above at each stage to maintain orientation and to assess the path of my argument.

PERSONHOOD AND DEMENTIA

There is much discussion of, and even more claim to, person-centred care in dementia care practice. Residential facilities, day care organisations, home care services and even government policy and guidance tie themselves into the discourse of 'person-centred-ness'. While this discourse has undoubtedly led to improvements in practice, it has, to my mind, led to some unfortunate, unforeseen and possibly unacknowledged problems.

Much of the discourse of person-centred care focuses on seeing the 'person behind the dementia'; in Kitwood's terms 'the person comes first' (1997a). Implicit in this way of thinking is the notion that the 'something' that is termed the 'person' is in some way distorted, changed, masked by the dementia, and it is that thing/person that needs to be protected from the deleterious impact of the disease and maintained in the face of its challenges. In practice persons are protected and maintained through a whole array of psycho-social interventions: reminiscence, life history, counselling, social networks and activities, and so on. These interventions act on two fronts: first, to ameliorate the deleterious effects of dementia; second, to defend the 'person' against the impact of dementia. These two related sets of interventions make sense within Kitwood's formulation of dementia in the following equation:

$$D = P + B + H + NI + SP$$

where D = dementia, P = personality, B = biography, H = health, NI = neurological impairment and SP = social psychology (see Kitwood 1997a).

The underlying logic here is that the dementia can be managed through the management of P, B, H, NI and SP. As a result the individual is incorporated into a number of 'systems' that are designed to manage (humanely) these aspects of the self: for example, biography becomes the subject of life history, reminiscence, memory boxes and so on, each with their tailored activities, policies, procedures and personnel. The individual thus becomes the object of management across a number of fields of intervention – all in the name of person-centred care. In sociological terminology, the individual becomes increasingly subject to the system world (Habermas 1984, 1987) and increasingly removed from the lifeworld.

SYSTEM WORLD AND LIFEWORLD

The literature on dementia care, theory and practice is surprisingly lacking in sociological theory – even Innes' text (2009), which purports to address dementia studies and the social sciences, is acutely devoid of social theory and critique. Although Kitwood made some attempt in his early writings to relate dementia to wider sociological ideas through the relations between psychobiography and capitalism (Kitwood 1990), these more overtly political pathways were later abandoned (Baldwin and Capstick 2007). Some authors, however, have attempted to draw on sociological theory – for example Small, Froggatt and Downs (2007). In their discussion of dementia care, Small *et al.* draw on Habermas' distinction between the system world and the life world. For Habermas (1984, 1987) the system world is a rationalised world in which the person is reduced to 'part of the "machinery" by which the system does what it does' (Frank undated). The lifeworld both stands in contrast to this and resists the encroachment of the system world, though the system world acts to colonise the lifeworld through imposing its logic on aspects of the lifeworld – for example care *management*, or the process and experience of dying (Small *et al.* 2007). The machinery in our case here refers to the system of interdependent and overlapping networks of management aimed at maintaining the person behind the dementia. The problem here, however, is that by focusing on this essentialist self, the uniqueness of the present 'person with dementia' is lost, in favour of a preferable idealised past when the person was intact.

While the above might sound harsh and unfair to the thousands of caring, hard-working and well-intentioned people involved in dementia care, I would ask you to hold your indignation while I take a short diversion before returning to complete my argument. This diversion will take us into the province of ethics, both as an example of what I am suggesting above and as an expansion of my argument.

PERSONHOOD AS THE OBJECT/SUBJECT OF ETHICS

It is interesting to note that the dominant framework in health care and bio-ethics, principlism, leaves little room for the notion of personhood as the object/subject of ethical reflection. Within this framework, developed by Beauchamp and Childress (2001), bioethical reflection, based on the four principles of autonomy, beneficence, non-maleficence and justice, becomes a tool wielded as a means to making defensible health care decisions. The framework itself has little, if anything, to say about the decision-makers, the individual about/for/with whom the decision is being made, the relationships between actors in the situation and the relationships between decisions over time or longer-term goals (or at least longer-term goals that are not already framed within the principlist framework, such as maintaining autonomy). In this way, the principlist framework becomes abstracted from the concrete situation: moral actors are, in some sense, replaceable by other moral actors who engage the principlist framework; ethical decisions become a function of the framework rather than the moral probity of the persons involved; the ethical encounter is more a decision-making process than a meeting, a dialogue between persons.

And it is this reduction of ethics to a subset of decision-making that exemplifies my argument above regarding the incorporation of the individual into the system world: within the principlist framework individuals become little more than carriers of a process of ethical decision-making. Let me explain: the proponents of principlism claim that the four principles (autonomy, beneficence, non-maleficence and justice) are universal, that is, while people may disagree because of individual beliefs or cultural practices, they may not disagree that the moral standards that underlie their beliefs:

- are simple, accessible and culturally neutral

- embrace a common set of moral commitments

- generate a common moral language; and

- cluster together a common set of moral issues.

In effect, within principlism, ethics is corralled within a decision-making structure bounded by the four principles. The four principles can thus be applied regardless of who is applying them, in what situations the principles are being applied and to whom the principles are being applied. Individual actors, according to this manner of ethical reasoning, are substitutable – it does not matter if A or B applies the principles to C, D or E in situations X, Y or Z, as the principles are universal, accessible, culturally neutral and generate a common language and a common set of moral issues. Whoever applies the principles to whomsoever in whatever situation, the process remains the same – and the same decision should, ideally, be made. This substitutability is only possible because the individuality and the relationships of those involved in the process are removed from the purview of ethical consideration by attributing a priori precedence to the four principles. Such a move, from the focus on the Other to the focus on principles 'reduc[ing] the Other who calls me as a unique self in the face-to-face to a set of a priori moral principles is a violence to her alterity' (Robbins 2000). In this way ethical decision-making becomes systematised – brought into the system world of efficiency, calculability and technical rationality: a sort of 'McDonaldisation' of ethics (Ritzer 2004).

And so I return to my argument regarding the system versus the lifeworld. In its systemisation of ethics, principlism colonises the lifeworld by imposing on relationships an abstracted rationality of how people should act toward one another. This systematisation limits the ways individuals can relate ethically toward one another and thus impoverishes ethical reasoning. In this I am, quite unusually, in agreement with Harris when he says that the universal application of principlism would 'lead to sterility and uniformity of approach of a quite mind-bogglingly boring kind' (Harris 2003, p.303).

DEVELOPING A PERSON-CENTRED ETHIC

So, if principlism is inadequate to the task of maintaining personhood, what might be an alternative path? We can, I think, find possibilities in the work of Buber (1958) and Levinas (1961) which, when fused with the insights from narrative theorists and philosophers such as Deleuze and Guattari (1972), provide avenues worth exploring. This is not to say that I can here present a fully formulated ethical framework – indeed this would in some ways be to go against the argument that I will be making. I hope, however, to point to possibilities, pathways that might help us think about how we relate to each other, and in particular how we might relate to persons living with dementia.

Buber

My starting point in this stage of my argument is Buber's notion of the I–Thou relationship (Buber 1958). For Buber the I–Thou relationship stands in contrast to the I–It relationship. The latter is a relationship between subject and object which involves a separation and detachment from that object. In contrast the I–Thou relationship is a relationship between two subjects, a relationship that affirms the Other through the act of choosing to relate in this way. The I–Thou relationship is one that is not mediated through any system of ideas or frameworks but relies on the direct contact of persons in their surprising uniqueness.

Kitwood drew on Buber when putting forward his view of personhood in dementia (1997a). For Kitwood, it was important that we look behind the dementia to the person – in the words of the subtitle of his most famous book, 'the person comes first'. Personhood, in Kitwood's view, was 'a standing or status that is bestowed upon one human being, by others, in the context of relationship and social being' (1997a, p.8). The advantages of this approach over that of the standard paradigm (that personhood is founded on essentialist traits, attributes or characteristics (Baldwin and Capstick 2007)) are that it is dynamic and relational.

Relating to another as 'Thou' necessitated, for Kitwood, a respect for the uniqueness and individuality of that person, being open to surprise and engagement in dialogue with no distant purpose, explicit or otherwise. Kitwood's interpretation of Buber was that to be a person is to be addressed as Thou (Kitwood 1997c).

However, Kitwood stepped back from realising the full implications of Buber's conceptualisation of the I–Thou relationship. For Buber, I–Thou relationships between individuals are founded on the more fundamental I–Thou relationship between the individual and God. Kitwood attempts to utilise Buber's philosophy to support his (Kitwood's) own humanistic stance and, while Kitwood and Buber are in alignment in the view that persons are not the objects for some distant goal, in Kitwood's work this is more a reflection of a Kantian ethic (of treating people as ends in themselves rather than means to one's own ends) than fidelity to Buber's I–Thou relationship. The difficulty for Kitwood was that, having abandoned his Christian faith and resigning his orders, he wanted to keep the foundational nature of Buber's I–Thou relationship without having the philosophical resources to do so.

Levinas

While I am not averse to Buber's overtly theological stance, I do not think it essential to the maintenance of a foundational stance toward the I–Thou relationship. The philosophical resources for this can, I think, be found in the work of Emmanuel Levinas (Levinas 1961). For Levinas, when the Self is faced with the presence of the Other, the Self's egoistic spontaneity, power and freedom is called into question. The Self is no longer in unique possession of the world and it is called to respond to the Other. This call to respond to what Levinas calls 'the Face' takes the shape of responsibility and obligation toward the Other in all her radical Otherness ('alterity', in Levinas' terminology). It is, according to Levinas, in responding to the Face that we become human. In this way ethics, the I–Thou relationship between the Self and Other, unmediated by a priori principles, theories, ideas, prejudices, desire to control, and so on, precedes ontology. In other words, it is in responding to the Face of the Other that we *become* human – and this is the foundation on which it is possible to build a truly person-centred ethic.

Deleuze and Guattari

I want now to take up this theme of 'becoming' as a fundamental part of what it means to be human. For Levinas it is in responding to the Face of the Other (that is, taking infinite responsibility for our relationship with the Other) that we become human. This becoming can only be an ongoing process, not a once-and-for-all event, for we are forever called upon to respond in uniquely existential ways to Others. This permanent *becoming* resonates, I think, with what Deleuze and Guattari (1972) term 'lines of flight' and the ongoing flux of de-territorialisation and re-territorialisation. To understand this way of thinking it is necessary to understand the person not as a fixed entity but as a being in process or as a multiplicity. A multiplicity is defined by a 'line of flight' along which it changes in nature through its connections with other multiplicities. Personhood is thus fluid, unstable, vulnerable to being re-territorialised, 'colonised' in Habermas' terminology (1984, 1987) by the system world but ever resistant through its response to the Face, the Other.

RECAPITULATION

Before moving on I think it may be wise to recapitulate. We have covered some complex ideas in the pursuit of the foundations of a person-centred ethic and, while what follows is somewhat less complex, it is important that the foundations are understood. Those who think I am being overly protective of my reader (or even patronising, though I do not mean to be) may skip ahead to the next section.

My argument to this point is that current thinking in person-centred care implies an essentialist view of the person: that is that there is something stable and intrinsic about individuals which should be maintained and promoted in the face of challenges such as that posed by the onset and progression of dementia. This essentialism facilitates the individual becoming an object of management with personality, health, biography, neurological impairment and social psychology all falling within the purview of expert systems within the logic of the system world. I illustrated this, and developed my argument through the example of principlism, the dominant framework in healthcare ethics, indicating how abstract, instrumental rationality has superseded direct, personal engagement and responsibility between autonomous moral actors.

Opposed to this, I drew on the work of Buber, in particular the I–Thou relationship, and found a non-theological foundation for this way of thinking and relating in Levinas' concept of the Face. With Levinas I suggested that it is in responding to the Face of the Other that we ourselves become human, and that this becoming is the very source of personhood. Becoming, following a line of flight, in the terminology of Deleuze and Guattari, involves ever-changing connections with others. Personhood is thus fluid, unstable and vulnerable to colonisation by the system world (in Habermasian terms) or re-territorialisation (in Deleuzean/Guattarian terms).

My contention – and to this I now turn – is that this view of personhood requires a different form of ethics, one that focuses on personhood as a process of becoming and has relationality at its heart.

PERSONALISM

I want to start this section of my argument with a discussion of personalism, an ethical framework emerging out of Catholicism (though not, I think, inextricably linked with it), which seeks to place personhood at the centre of ethical thinking. In personalism, being human and personhood are virtually synonymous. Personhood is an attribute or status of every human being, regardless of capacity, characteristics or ability. This personalist approach has, according to Palazzini (1994), four fundamental principles:

- the fundamental value of human life (by which Palazzini means body, mind and soul, not just physical life)

- totality or therapeutic value, that is that the totality of life, not just local considerations, be accounted for in making decisions

- freedom and responsibility, by which he means that freedom lies in making responsible choices

- sociality and assistance which centres on the view that the life and health of society are promoted through the health and life of every individual, and that assistance is provided to whomsoever needs help and support.

We can see that this framework takes account of the relational nature of being human, the inter-dependencies within which we all live, and has a sense of human flourishing through a concern for physical-psychological-spiritual complementarity and wholeness, and the placement of the individual within a network of social rights, responsibilities and mutuality.

Some of these themes were taken up by Schotsmans (1999), who argues that the personalist approach focuses on (1) the uniqueness of individuals, in (2) their relational and intersubjective milieux, linked by (3) the social bonds of communication and solidarity. These three features of personalism, for Schotsmans, provide a basis for moral action:

> With these three fundamental value orientations in mind we can articulate a moral criterion, with a personalist meaning: we say that an act is morally good if it serves the humanum or human dignity, that is if it in truth is beneficial to the human person adequately considered in these three basic value-orientations (dimensions and relationships): uniqueness, relational commitment and solidarity. (Schotsmans 1999, p.19)

In the above description of personalism we can trace resonances of both Buber and Levinas: there is a sense of becoming in its commitment to human flourishing; there is a commitment to responsibility to the Other, and a sense that our own wellbeing is bound up with that commitment and responsibility; and there is an acknowledgement of difference, the uniqueness of individuals. So far, so good. What it lacks, however, is a sense of the trajectory of an individual life, the navigation by an individual through time and place and the meanings attributed to those events and characters met along the way. In other words, personalism is not embedded within an experiential framework which helps us make sense of our lives. That experiential framework is found, I believe, in the notion of narrative, and it is to this we now turn.

NARRATIVE

The ubiquity of narrative seems to have done little to help define or clarify what is meant by terms such as 'the narrative self', a term that seems to have gained currency in recent years. Does the term 'the narrative self' mean that we understand who we are through the stories we tell (and the stories that others tell about us), a sort of window on our own experiential world? Or does it mean we construct who we are through the stories we tell (and stories that are told about us)? I place myself in the latter, constructivist camp, identifiable with the works of authors such as Jerome Bruner (1987, 1990), Alasdair MacIntyre (1985) and Charles Taylor (1989): we are who we are because of the stories we tell, are bound to, incorporated within, imagine, and so on (as opposed to telling the stories we tell because of who we are).

Let me start with MacIntyre. For MacIntyre the individual is embedded within its own history and the larger and longer histories of traditions. These histories make our lives intelligible and serve to promote what MacIntyre calls 'narrative unity'. Promoting and preserving that narrative unity is the task of the good life. This leads us back to Buber (1958) who wrote that the I–Thou relationship is founded in the unity of being. I am suggesting here that MacIntyre's narrative unity can be seen as akin to Buber's unity of being, which fosters the desired I–Thou relationship. In promoting narrative unity (the coherence of an individual life and the alignment of that life with the longer and larger narratives of tradition) we promote the ethical encounter that is the I–Thou relationship.

These longer and larger narratives of tradition can, in turn, be seen as akin to Taylor's 'web of interlocutions' – that is:

> one cannot be a self on one's own. I am a self only in relation to certain interlocutors: in one way in relation to those conversation partners who were essential to my achieving self-definition; in another in relation to those who are now crucial to my continuing grasp of languages and self-understanding – and, of course, these classes may develop. A self exists only within what I call 'webs of interlocution'. It is this original situation which gives its sense to our concept of 'identity', offering an answer to the question of who I am through a definition of where I am speaking from and to whom. The full definition of someone's identity thus usually involves not only his stand on moral and spiritual matters but also some reference to a defining community. (Taylor 1989, p.36)

These defining communities are multifarious and overlapping. Narrative traditions need not be coercive or limiting but appreciative of individual uniqueness and can allow for reconfigurations of traditional narratives within individual lives. Hence we can celebrate the narrative configurations expressed in queer and crip theory – that is, theories around how bodies, pleasures and identities are expressed and rendered through narrative as normal, deviant or even abject (McRuer 2006) – as unsettling of our traditional and normative narratives.

Of course, narrative traditions can be limiting; for example, stories of dementia used to be ones of loss and decline, but there are now an increasing number of dementia narratives stressing how to live positively with dementia. While this is an improvement, just as in Plummer's work on sexuality (1995) or Muncey's work on teenage pregnancy (2005), some dementia stories have yet to find a voice, namely the stories of the benefits and pleasures that dementia might bring.

Now, before I am silenced by howls of approbation or derision for suggesting this (and I have to confess that even I feel uneasy in writing this, indicating just how deeply ingrained meta-narratives of dementia are), I have interviewed carers who report that their relatives are more relaxed, less anxious now that they have dementia. One carer reported that her mother was now finding great pleasure in her great-grandchild (whereas previously her mother had little time for children), and it is said of William Penn, the Quaker, that developing dementia was God's way of allowing him to rest. Indeed, Kitwood at one point suggested that dementia might in some circumstances prompt personal growth (Kitwood 1995).

Each of these, admittedly small, examples of benefit and pleasure are flickers of alternative narratives that just might be waiting to be heard. As such these stories throw into question, or at least have the potential to throw into question, our assumptions about normalcy, in that they deviate both from the norm of cognitive intactness and from the norm of dementia stories of either loss or fortitude. But that is the glory of narrative – the uniqueness of individuals can find expression in a narrative unity, supported by a community or tradition, that allows for becoming (remember, lines of flight?) and resists colonisation and re-territorialisation by the system world.

CONCLUDING REMARKS

All of this has profound implications for dementia care, for if we jettison the essentialist version of personhood we can then explore the uniqueness of individuals in terms of how their multiplicitous personhood is constituted through their connections with other multiplicities, how that personhood is changing, becoming. This processual view of personhood does not require management in the form of standardised bio-psycho-social interventions but an imaginative response to the Other in his or her radical alterity. We cannot in advance say what maintaining/promoting personhood means (though it is certainly not the attempt to recapture something that used to be). It lies in the surprise of the I–Thou relationship where we each become human by responding to the presence of the Other. This is more the response of the artist than the clinician, and more Jackson Pollock than Norman Rockwell.

CHAPTER 18

A Situated Embodied View of the Person with Dementia

Where Does the Spiritual Come In?

Julian C. Hughes

INTRODUCTION

The question I wish to address is whether the notion of spirituality is negotiable. I shall relate this to dementia. I want to move from questions about normativity to questions about existence. I shall largely be offering a philosophical exploration of the justification for including spirituality amongst the ways that we think when we think of people with dementia. I hope these somewhat opaque comments will become clearer. Let me start by sketching the background to the question.

It has become commonplace for healthcare workers to speak in terms of the biopsychosocial model of disease (Engel 1980). In addition, we now have the model of palliative care, which includes the idea that we should pay attention not only to the biological, psychological and social, but also to the spiritual needs of our patients (World Health Organization 2010). Palliative care is increasingly seen as relevant to dementia, not just at the end of life, but from the time of diagnosis to beyond death, since attention must also be paid to bereavement (Hughes 2006). So the emergence of palliative care as a model for dementia suggests the importance of spirituality in our thinking about people with dementia. In this chapter, my aim is to outline some philosophical grounds for an emphasis on spirituality in connection with dementia. In so doing, I am also lending support to the idea that we should be using the model of palliative care for people with dementia. But I am doing this in a particular way, because my suggestion is not that the model of palliative care is the only model on the street. Indeed, I see palliative care in the context of a broader model of supportive care as the appropriate paradigm (Hughes, Lloyd-Williams and Sachs 2010). What I am commending is precisely the idea of a *broad* model: it is the breadth that is key, not the name of the model. A question underlying some of my discussion will be to do with whether it makes sense to speak of limits to the model. Is it rational to think of boundaries to our models of dementia?

But the other important and ubiquitous model in connection with dementia is that of person-centred care, made famous by Tom Kitwood (1997a). In the next section, I shall discuss how we should characterize the notion of personhood. The question and the task is the same: can we pin down what it is to be a person (are there boundaries or limits to this notion)? Or perhaps there should be no limits (in a sense) to what a person might be. To my way of thinking, personhood is central to any of our models for understanding dementia. What we have to say about personhood will determine how we should think of dementia (i.e. the models we might use). So the motivation for the argument I sketch here is to do with whether spirituality is a non-negotiable ingredient of personhood. I think it is; and later I shall gesture at some practical implications of this for dementia care.

THE SEA VIEW

There has been a tendency in philosophical writings about dementia to define personhood in a limited way. Thus questions can be asked such as: is the person who made the advance directive the same person as the one who now has severe dementia, to whom the advance directive should be applied (if it is the same person)? If, for instance, personhood is tied tightly to memory, then it follows that personhood is lost as memory is lost. A corollary of this train of thought is that the individual with severe dementia is no longer a person at all. Such ideas can be linked to the names of philosophers such as John Locke and Derek Parfit; these ideas need not detain us (but see Hughes, Louw and Sabat 2006), except to note that the effect is to limit the notion of personhood, to tie it tightly to the idea of a particular type of memory. The characterization of a person as a *situated embodied agent* (the SEA view) is intended to counteract such limited views of what might constitute personhood (Hughes 2001).

First, then, a person is *situated*. In other words, we are neither islands nor discrete atoms, but are interconnected and mutually dependent beings. We are situated in families or at least in family histories. At a minimum we are located in our own personal histories, or narratives, which have multiple layers and are typically (if not inevitably) co-authored or co-constructed. But we are also situated in a social and cultural context, as well as in a legal system with its own moral underpinnings as part of a political structure to which we contribute, more or less.

Second, we are *embodied*. We cannot escape our biology and the consequences of it. We are, however, more than just bodies, because our bodies are more than *just* our bodies! It is our bodies that show our mental and emotional lives. We are, to use the phrase derived from the philosopher Maurice Merleau-Ponty, body subjects (Matthews 2002); in other words, our subjectivity is embodied (Kontos 2004). Or, as Ludwig Wittgenstein (1968) put it: 'The human body is the best picture of the human soul' (p.178).

Finally, we are *agents*: we act on the world, make decisions, exert an influence. Or, at least, we have in our nature the potential to do these things, whether or not we actually do them. This brings out another aspect of this characterization of the person, which is that the components do not appear in isolation. For we are situated agents, and we are situated in a bodily form. So, even if I am not acting as an agent because I have lost some of my agentive skills, I am situated in a history in which I have been or will be an agent; and even if (at the extreme) this is not true (because I am in an irreversible coma, say), my embodiment is such that agentive powers are *characteristic* of my being this sort of individual. It is the potential derived from being situated thus – as the type of being that is typically agentive – that helps to characterize me as a person. Hence, on my view, to be a person is to be a situated embodied agent.

THE SPIRITUAL AND THE TRANSCENDENT

Before proceeding with my argument, I need to give an account of spirituality. In discussing the notion of 'meaning in life', Sapp (2010) uses the suggestion that spirituality is seen

> as speaking of that which gives one a sense of *connectedness* – to oneself, to others, to the natural world, and to that which transcends all of these categories, a transpersonal source of power commonly called the sacred, the divine, or God, what Twelve-Step Programs refer to as a 'Higher Power', however conceived by a given individual…
>
> Spirituality, therefore, is often especially associated with questions about finding 'meaning' and 'purpose' in human existence, particularly in the last stage of a person's life when one's impending death renders unavoidable the question of what one's life has meant. (Sapp 2010, p.200)

I want to focus particularly on the idea that spirituality has something to do with transcendence.

This seems right. Whatever else it is, 'spirit' cannot refer to something worldly in the sense of something physically present. It may be immanent in the world, but it is not part of the physical furniture. Our only access to the spiritual is through worldly things, whether these are sunsets or human smiles, so it is part of the world. The spiritual dwells within a sunset or a smile, perhaps – it is immanent in this sense – but it is transcendent too, in that it goes beyond the physical features of the sunset or smile. The 'going beyond' is a key feature of the notion of 'spirit' that I wish to capture, which is to say that I want to point to the transcendent as a defining feature of what spirituality is about. But this entails that I do not fully *know* what it is that I am pointing at: it is 'beyond' – there is something mysterious about the spirit. Spirituality is a manifestation of our openness to mystery.

NORMATIVE CONSTRAINTS

Sapp's (2010) discussion of spirituality also linked it to meaning: the meaning of our lives. But I want to use this to take us back to what it is to be a person. One of the characteristics of human persons is that we can mean things. We have language, or at least we are situated in a form of life that involves language and entails meaning. The argument that I now wish to put forward concerns the nature of meaning. In brief, I want to say that meaning is normative. In other words, if I say that the clouds are moving swiftly towards the Town Moor, for this to have meaning, it must be the case (roughly speaking) that there are such things as clouds that can move swiftly towards a place recognized as the Town Moor. My mental state of meaning 'this' when I say 'that' is normatively constrained in the sense that something in the world has to be one way rather than another. Similarly, for me to remember, certain things must be the case. This is a general property of mental states that philosophers call intentionality, which is a technical term used to suggest *aboutness* or *ofness*. In other words, when I mean, understand, remember, and so on, my meaning is *about* something, my understanding and memory are *of* something. These types of mental state, for them to be the mental states that they are, are normatively constrained by the world being this way rather than that. Normativity is a matter of there being criteria of correctness. Understanding normativity has been a major endeavour in philosophy of thought and language. How do we account for normativity?

Philosophers have pursued various accounts (Luntley 2003). At this point it is necessary to introduce a further technical term from philosophy, because such accounts of normativity can often be described as transcendental. This is a sense associated with the writings of Immanuel Kant. A transcendental argument is one that looks at the preconditions for something. Space and time are preconditions for the existence of the external world. So, too, there is a transcendental account to be given of normativity. It suggests that normativity is embedded in human worldly practices – namely the practices of understanding, meaning, memory and the like – for these to be the practices that they are. When we learn to understand something, we learn a practice in which the criteria of correctness are embedded: they are not added subsequently; they are not elsewhere. This would not be an example of meaning '*x*' if the normative constraints (that make it '*x*' rather than '*y*') were not *part of what it is* to mean anything. We can say that normativity is immanent to the practices. A condition for the possibility of my meaning '*x*' is that it is inherent to the notion of meaning something that, when I do, I demonstrate a practice, part and parcel of which is the normatively constrained feature that only *this* will do. Calling this a transcendental argument simply shows us the form of the argument: from something that is not argued, that meaning '*x*' means just this (*x*), we look to the conditions for the possibility that this is so, and we conclude that the practice of meaning is inherently normative (otherwise the concept of meaning loses its grip on the world).

GOING QUIET?

This may seem all very well, but what is the connection with spirituality? Well, first, this argument can be taken as supportive of the SEA view of the person. The argument about intentional mental states shows how our inner worlds, our subjectivity, must inherently (at a conceptual level) involve the world. These mental states (meaning, remembering, understanding, and so on) as a transcendental feature are normatively constrained. To be able to mean or understand something is to be able to participate in a worldly practice for which the criteria of correctness have been grasped as part of learning the practice. Being a human person, therefore, being able to demonstrate characteristic patterns of human practice, being minded, is to engage with the world in a particular manner. It is to be situated in the world and agentive in the sense that it requires doing, that is: the ability to participate in typically human practices in a human person sort of way (e.g. bodily).

Second, the argument that normativity resides in worldly human practices is intended to end the discussion, in that normativity cannot be explained further. It makes no sense to ask what ensures the normativity in the practices themselves; normativity is just a feature of the practice: it is what makes it the practice that it is. As far as the argument in debates about thought and language go, this is the point where some philosophers commend the idea of quietism: nothing further can be said by way of justification; we simply have the worldly practices.

But need the conversation stop here? Some philosophers argue against quietism, for instance saying that it is not *just* that we have practices, they are justified by the community adopting them. This is akin to a social constructionist line of thought: the criteria of correctness come from community use. We construct meaning. Another approach is the platonic one: there is a platonic heaven in which meanings are laid down. When we use a word with meaning, on this view, we make contact correctly with its form in the transcendental platonic realm. So, to put it crudely (and to ignore other options or the subtleties of the arguments), meanings are either made up by us here on earth or they reside in some sort of heaven.

GOING BROAD

But such counter-arguments to quietism are not my concern. I wish to bring back into play elements from my earlier discussion. First, we are situated and, as we saw, this implies a broad view. Indeed, it is uncircumscribable. There are always further possibilities for human beings. To be humanly situated is always to have different ways *to be* in the world. Second, I want to return to the technical notion of a transcendental argument. This is where the argument looks at the preconditions: the conditions for the possibility of such and such being the case. With these two elements in mind we can now ask a question that goes beyond the debates about meaning in the philosophy of thought and language: what are the conditions for the possibility of there being the human worldly practices that are constitutive of meaning?

The thing to note is that this is a question about the world. OK, we might say, there are no further justifications within the world, but does not the world itself raise a question? Again the philosophical arguments must necessarily be brief. We have already encountered Kant's argument that space and time are preconditions, in fact a priori notions, that make the experience of the world possible. But space and time are also part of our worldly experience. There is a further question that can be raised about the conditions for the possibility of *any* worldly practices or experiences. Furthermore, this links to our experience of being situated. For, I am situated in an expanding field. There is my personal history, but this is embedded in my family history, which is embedded in a cultural and social history, which involves laws and political systems, and so on. But the point I made earlier was that the '...and so on' cannot be circumscribed. I am also situated in a world of art, which has many forms, and sport, and other examples of human endurance and courage, as well as being a part of the natural world, where what is now happening in the rainforests of Brazil and the factories of China and the nuclear reprocessing plant at Sellafield can all impinge on my existence or being-in-the-world. In which case, however, can it also be said that I am situated in a spiritual realm too?

So we have two questions and a statement. The first question is: what are the conditions for the possibility of there being *any* human worldly practices, that is, any world at all? The statement is: we are situated in expanding domains. The second question is: does it make sense to think that we are also situated in a spiritual domain? Well, it is open to a sceptic to deny that the expansion of the domains in which we are situated needs to encompass the spiritual, and therefore the answer to the second question will be negative. Or, being more charitable, the sceptic might allow that individuals can see themselves as situated in a spiritual field if they are so inclined, a perception that should be accepted and (charitably) respected – but in which case, the notion of spirituality is negotiable. My view, however, is that spirituality is a non-negotiable aspect of our being-in-the-world.

The reason is the first question. Our being in the world, our having worldly practices in which normativity inheres, raises a question. It is a question that points beyond the world; in this sense it is transcendental. And the key point is not about the answer; it is about the rationality of the question. If we can raise questions within the world, questions that will be in one way or another about our being, why does not *being itself* raise a question? Why should our questioning be closed down before we ask the question about being (the existence of the world) itself? That question, which is transcendental (it is looking for the conditions for the possibility of there being anything at all), also points towards something that must be transcendental, that is, something beyond the world. In which case the question points in the direction of what I was inclined to call the spiritual realm, which is mysterious. And I am saying that the mystery of the spiritual arises in response to the rationality of the question. We move from things being thus and so, the normativity that characterizes intentional mental states, to a radical question about the existence of the world. As Wittgenstein (1974) put it: 'It is not *how* things are in the world that is mystical, but *that* it exists' (§6.44).

So, for me, spirituality is a matter of seeing that the world raises a question that points at a mystery. Of course, this might mean that my notion of spirituality is different from that of some others. Spirituality is not, on my view, just an emotional state, even if contemplation of the mystery of the world is likely to induce particular human reactions. What we do about our spirituality is a personal matter, which may or may not include specific religious observances. But, on my view, because the question ineluctably arises, spirituality is non-negotiable. Failure to see the mystery is a failure in human flourishing.[1]

CONCLUSION

So spirituality is part and parcel of what it is to be a person, qua human being in the world. Therefore, our models of dementia – person-centred, palliative, supportive – must be broad enough to encompass spirituality, not as an add-on, but as a fundamental feature. If part of my personhood is my spirituality, then you can help to maintain my personhood (in part at least) by paying attention to my spiritual needs. People with dementia, even in the severer stages, respond to rituals and familiar prayers (Allen and Coleman 2006). But the deeper need, for they may *not* respond, is for the person not to be thought of as an individual autonomous agent, but as a situated embodied agent: one who is interconnected in an interdependent world (Allen and Coleman 2006; Sapp 2010). The non-negotiable standing of the spiritual realm means that, even in the absence of religious belief, the mystery that is central to our being-in-the-world should engender a sense of wonder at the importance of the person. Beings of this type, just on account of our situatedness together, must be afforded the solicitude that Heidegger regarded as intrinsic to our typical stance in the human world of *Being-with* (Heidegger 1962). Spirituality in dementia often focuses on the carers, who are, after all, those who are best placed to maintain the person's standing as someone of moral worth and dignity.

> And as the 'things of this world', which the modern world has come to rely upon for meaning, necessarily diminish in importance and begin to disappear, if carers for persons with dementia are to maintain hope and a sense of the meaningfulness of life, as is the case with those for whom they care, the source of that hope and meaning must increasingly be that which transcends the earthly dimension, namely, the things of the spirit. (Sapp 2010, p.206)

The way in which close (usually family) carers, who so often suffer significant stress, can also describe a sense of moral growth despite their experiences is testimony to the possibility that something transcendent can occur in the context of advanced dementia. But even if the person with dementia and the carer had or have no sense of the spiritual, it remains true that care itself – 'solicitude' in Heidegger's terminology – must be understood in the context of the broader view. According to this view, our ways of understanding dementia and the possibilities of care must be unbounded. Spirituality is a way of breaking down the boundaries of thought and language that otherwise confine our ways of both Being and Being-with in dementia.

NOTE

1. Anyone familiar with Herbert McCabe's essay 'Creation' will recognize my line of argument in the latter part of this chapter (see McCabe 1987, pp.2–9). I have bent the argument to my own purposes, but I would strongly recommend McCabe's essay to anyone looking for a good argument for the existence of God. I am happy to acknowledge the tremendous debt I feel to the late Father McCabe.

THE CONTRIBUTORS

Brian Allen is Chaplaincy Team Leader, Northumberland, Tyne and Wear NHS Foundation Trust. He has trained staff in spiritual and cultural awareness, person-centred care of people with dementia and mindfulness-based approaches for caring for ourselves and others. He managed the Dementia Projects of the Christian Council on Ageing.

Clive Baldwin is Senior Lecturer in Social Work (Mental Health) at the University of Bradford. Prior to this he undertook post-doctoral research at ETHOX at the University of Oxford on ethical issues facing family carers of relatives with dementia and then worked at the Bradford Dementia Group, coordinating the MSc in Dementia Studies.

Padmaprabha Dalby is a consultant clinical psychologist who specialises in working with older people. She qualified in her profession in 1993 and currently leads psychological and therapy services for older people in Sussex Partnership NHS Foundation Trust. In 2009, she completed a clinical psychology doctorate on the theme of spirituality and older people, which included the research described in this book. Padmaprabha has been committed to a Buddhist lifestyle for 25 years and is interested in finding spiritual significance and meaning in the experience of everyday life.

Malcolm Goldsmith was ordained in the Church of England almost 50 years ago and is now retired. He has been a chaplain to a hospice and a research fellow at the Dementia Services Development Centre in Stirling, and spent many years in parish ministry. He has lectured and written widely on issues related to ageing in general and to dementia in particular.

Margaret Goodall is currently Chaplaincy Advisor for Methodist Homes for the Aged Care Group, having previously been chaplain in a dementia care home for 15 years. She is now completing her Professional Doctorate with Chester University on spirituality and dementia. A Methodist minister living in Milton Keynes, she is also Chair of the Dementia Working Group for the Christian Council on Ageing. Margaret has contributed to several books on environmental theology and ageing and dementia.

Paul Green trained as a mental health nurse at the University of Wales, Bangor (1996–1999) and gained extensive experience in day services for older people and as a liaison nurse for people with dementia before training as a cognitive behavioural psychotherapist at the University of Huddersfield (2009–2010). He also completed degrees in health and social care (Open University 2003) and psychosocial interventions (Leeds Metropolitan University 2008). Paul has published a number of papers in professional journals and continues to maintain his interest in adapting CBT to meet the needs of older people as a cognitive behavioural psychotherapist employed by the Kirklees Primary Care Psychological Therapies Service. He is on the editorial board of *CBT Today* and occasionally contributes articles to the arts pages of *The Friend*. Paul lives in West Yorkshire with his wife, Emma.

Gaynor Hammond is a Baptist minister. Her background is in nursing and for seven years she was in post as the Dementia Project Worker for Faith in Elderly People, Leeds. For the past 12 years she has been in post as Regional Tutor for Northern Baptist College and with South Parade Baptist Church in Leeds.

Julian C. Hughes is a consultant in old age psychiatry based at North Tyneside General Hospital. He is honorary Professor of Philosophy of Ageing at the Institute for Ageing and Health, Newcastle University. His most recent, co-edited, book is *Supportive Care for the Person with Dementia* (Oxford University Press, 2010).

Albert Jewell is a retired Methodist minister and former Pastoral Director of MHA Care Group (Methodist Homes). He completed his PhD study of the sources of wellbeing in older Methodists in 2007 at the University of Wales, Bangor. He is vice-chair of the Christian Council on Ageing and edits its dementia newsletter. He is also editor of *Spirituality and Ageing* (1999) and *Ageing, Spirituality and Well-being* (2004), both published by Jessica Kingsley Publishers.

John Killick has been working with people with dementia for 16 years. He is interested especially in communication and creativity, and has written and spoken widely on these subjects. He is currently Writer in Residence for Alzheimer Scotland. His website is www.dementiapositive.co.uk.

Dr Murray Lloyd practised as a Consultant Physician in Extended Care for 40 years, passing through the fields of cardiology, rehabilitation, palliative care and, finally, aged care. He has created programmes for teaching communication to staff throughout his career and, in retirement since 2001, has particularly focused on the spiritual needs of older people.

Rev Prof Elizabeth MacKinlay AM is a registered nurse, a priest in the Anglican Church and the Director of the Centre for Ageing and Pastoral Studies at St Mark's National Theological Centre, Canberra. She is a Professor in the School of Theology, Charles Sturt University. Recently completed research includes *Finding Meaning in the Experience of Dementia: The Place of Spiritual Reminiscence Work*, an Australian Research Council project. Elizabeth was Chair of the ACT Ministerial Advisory Council on Ageing, her term ending in 2008. An active researcher and writer, she has presented many papers and workshops, including keynote addresses both nationally and internationally. One of her recent books, *Spiritual Growth and Care in the Fourth Age of Life* (2006), was winner of the Australasian Journal on Ageing (AJA) Book Award. Elizabeth is editor of the new book based on the CAPS 2008 conference, *Ageing and Spirituality across Faiths and Cultures* (2010), which follows soon after the release of the Japanese version of *Facilitating Spiritual Reminiscence in People with Dementia*.

Susan H. McFadden PhD is Professor of Psychology, University of Wisconsin Oshkosh. She received her doctorate in Psychology and Religion from Drew University in 1985 and has been active in both the American Society on Aging and the Gerontological Society of America, bringing together researchers and practitioners interested in religion, spirituality, and aging.

Harriet Mowat is Managing Director of Mowat Research. She works with universities and health and social care agencies to improve care of older people and attitudes to them. She lives near Inverness in Scotland with her husband and two labradors. Much of the thinking behind her research goes on while she is walking the dogs.

Wendy Shiels has been the Dementia and Palliative Care Coordinator of a large nursing home in Melbourne, Australia, since 2002. Formerly a family carer, she worked for many years with Alzheimer's Australia Victoria, is a 2001 Churchill Fellow and an experienced Dementia Care Mapper, and lectures and writes on caring for people who are living with dementia.

John Swinton holds the chair in Practical Theology and Pastoral Care at the University of Aberdeen, Scotland. He is also an honorary Professor at Aberdeen's Centre for Advanced Studies in Nursing. Professor Swinton worked as a registered nurse specialising in psychiatry and learning disabilities and also for a number of years as a community mental health chaplain. His areas of research include the relationship between spirituality and health and the theology and spirituality of disability. In 2004 he founded the Centre for Spirituality, Health and Disability at the University of Aberdeen (www.abdn.ac.uk/cshad). He is the author of *Spirituality in Mental Health: Rediscovering a Forgotten Dimension* (Jessica Kingsley Publishers, 2001) and *Resurrecting the Person* (Abingdon Press, 2000).

Marianne Talbot's parents both had dementia. For two years she chronicled the tears and laughter of caring in *Keeping Mum*, a blog written for Saga Magazine Online, due to become a book in 2011. Marianne is also Director of Studies in Philosophy at Oxford University's Department for Continuing Education.

Daphne Wallace practised psychiatry in the NHS from 1966 to 2000, serving as a consultant psychiatrist from 1979 to 2000 and continuing in psychotherapy practice until 2007. She has been involved in the development of the National Dementia Strategy and is currently co-chair of its implementation group. She is a member and former trustee of the Alzheimer's Society. A founder member of the Christian Council on Ageing Dementia Group, she was diagnosed with early vascular dementia in 2005.

REFERENCES

Adams, K., Hyde, B. and Woolley, R. (2008) *The Spiritual Dimension of Childhood*. London: Jessica Kingsley Publishers.

Adams, T. (1996) 'Kitwood's approach to dementia and dementia care: A critical but appreciative review.' *Journal of Advanced Nursing 23*, 5, 948–953.

Airey, J., Hammond, G., Kent, P. and Moffitt, L. (2002) *Frequently Asked Questions on Spirituality and Religion*. Derby: Christian Council on Ageing.

Alexopoulos, G.S. (2003) 'Clinical and biological interactions in affective and cognitive geriatric symptoms.' *American Journal of Psychiatry 160*, 811–814.

Allen, B. (2002) *Religious Practice and People with Dementia*. Derby: Christian Council on Ageing.

Allen, B. (2008) 'Dementia: Remembering the cost.' *Crucible, The Journal of Christian Social Ethics,* April–June.

Allen, B. (2010) 'Remembering the Cost: A Theological Reflection.' In J. Woodward (ed.) *Between Remembering and Forgetting*. London: Continuum Mobray.

Allen, F.B. and Coleman, P.G. (2006). 'Spiritual Perspectives on the Person with Dementia.' In J.C. Hughes, S.J. Louw and S.R. Sabat (eds) *Dementia: Mind, Meaning, and the Person*. Oxford: Oxford University Press.

Alzheimer's Society (2010). 'Singing for the Brain.' Available at www.alzheimers.org.uk/site/scripts/documents_info.php?documentID=760, accessed on 21 November 2010.

Antonowski, A. (1987) *Unravelling the Mystery of Health*. San Francisco, CA: Jossey-Bass Publishers.

Arthey, V. (1997). *Is Anyone There?* Derby: Christian Council on Ageing [DVD].

Baldwin, C. and Capstick, A. (2007) *Tom Kitwood on Dementia: A Reader and Critical Commentary*. Maidenhead: Open University Press.

Basting, A.D. (2008) *ArtCare: The Story of How an Arts Program Can Transform Long Term Care*. Milwaukee, WI: UWM Center on Aging and Community.

Basting, A.D. (2009) *Forget Memory: Creating Better Lives for People with Dementia*. Baltimore, MD: Johns Hopkins University Press.

BBC and Royal College of Nursing (1999) *When Your Heart Wants to Remember* [DVD]. No longer available.

Beard, R.L. (2004) 'In their voices: Identity preservation and experiences of Alzheimer's disease.' *Journal of Aging Studies 18*, 415–428.

Beauchamp, T.L. and Childress, J.F. (2001) *Principles of Biomedical Ethics*, fifth edition. New York: Oxford University Press.

Beck, A.T., Epstein, N., Brown, G. and Steer, R.A. (1988) 'An inventory for measuring clinical anxiety: Psychometric properties.' *Journal of Consulting and Clinical Psychology 56*, 6, 893–897.

Berger, P.L. (1997) *Redeeming Laughter: The Comic Dimension of Human Experience*. New York: Walter De Gruyter.

Besig, D. and Price, N. (1986) *As Long as I Have Music*. Delaware Water Gap, PA: Shawnee Press.

Board of Social Responsibility (1990) *Ageing*. London: Church House Publishing.

Boden, C. (1998) *Who Will I Be When I Die?* Pymble: Harper Collins Religious.

Brennan, A. (1990) 'Fragmented selves and the problem of ownership.' *Proceedings of the Aristotelian Society 90*, 143–158.

Brock, F. (2008) 'Houston Faith Communities Collaborate on Memory Care Day Centre.' In S.H. McFadden and C. Kozberg (eds) *Religion, Spirituality, and Meaning in Later Life. Generations 32*, 2, 42–43.

Bruner, J. (1987) 'Life as narrative.' *Social Research 54*, 1, 11–32.

Bruner, J. (1990) *Acts of Meaning.* Cambridge, MA: Harvard University Press.

Bryden, C. (2005) *Dancing with Dementia: My Story of Living Positively with Dementia.* London and Philadelphia, PA: Jessica Kingsley Publishers.

Bryden, C. and MacKinlay, E.B. (2002) 'Dementia – a spiritual journey towards the divine: A personal view of dementia.' *Journal of Religious Gerontology 13*, 3/4, 69–75

Bryden, C. and MacKinlay, E. (2008) 'Dementia: A Journey Inwards to a Spiritual Self.' In E. MacKinlay (ed.) *Ageing, Disability and Spirituality.* London and Philadelphia, PA: Jessica Kingsley Publishers..

Buber, M. (1958) *I and Thou* (transl. R. Gregor Smith). New York: Charles Scribner's Sons. First published (1923) as *Ich und Du.* Leipzig: Insel-Verlag.

Buber, M. (1970) *I and Thou* (transl. W. Kaufmann). New York: Charles Scribner's Sons. First published (1923) as *Ich und Du.* Leipzig: Insel-Verlag.

Buchanan, M. (2002) *Things Unseen: Living in Light of Forever.* Sisters, OR: Multnomah Publishers.

Campbell, A.V. (1985) *Paid to Care?* London: SPCK.

Campbell, D. (1997) *The Mozart Effect.* Rydalmere: Hodder and Stoughton.

Carter, S. (1963) 'I danced in the morning' ('Lord of the dance'). London: Stainer and Bell Ltd.

Cassidy, S. (1988) *Sharing the Darkness: The Spirituality of Caring.* London: Darton, Longman and Todd.

Castelo, D. (2009) *The Apathetic God: Exploring the Contemporary Relevance of Divine Impassibility.* London: Paternoster.

Chapman, A. and Killick, J. (1997) 'One to One: Towards a Deeper Level of Communication' [video cassette]. Stirling: University of Stirling.

Chardin, P. Teilhard de (1960) *Le Milieu Divin.* London: Collins.

Charlesworth, G.M. and Reichelt, F.K. (2004) 'Keeping conceptualisations simple: Examples with family carers of people with dementia.' *Behavioural and Cognitive Psychotherapy 32*, 4, 401–409.

Chatterjee, M. (1989) *The Concept of Spirituality.* New Delhi: Allied Publishers.

Cheston, R. and Bender, M. (2003) *Understanding Dementia: The Man with the Worried Eyes.* London and Philadelphia, PA: Jessica Kingsley Publishers.

Chew-Graham, C., Baldwin, R. and Burns, A. (2004) 'Treating depression in later life.' *British Medical Journal 329*, 181–182.

Chittister, J. (2003) *Scarred by Struggle, Transformed by Hope.* Grand Rapids, MI: Wm Eerdmans Publishing Co.

Chopra, M.P., Sullivan, J.R., Feldman, Z., Landes, R.D. and Beck, C. (2008) 'Self, collateral and clinician assessment of depression in persons with cognitive impairment.' *Aging and Mental Health 12*, 6, 675–683.

Clare, L., Rowlands, J., Bruce, E., Surr, C. and Downs, M. (2008) 'The experience of living with dementia in residential care: An interpretative phenomenological analysis.' *The Gerontologist 48*, 6, 711–720.

Clarke, R. (2010) 'State of Grace.' In L. Whitman (ed.) *Telling Tales about Dementia: Experiences of Caring.* London and Philadelphia, PA: Jessica Kingsley Publishers.

Clinebell, H. (1996) *Well Being.* Quezon City, Philippines: Kadena Books.

Cobb, M. (2005) *The Hospital Chaplain's Handbook: A Guide for Good Practice.* Norwich: Canterbury Press.

Cohen, G. (2000) *The Creative Age: Awakening Human Potential.* San Francisco, CA: Harper Collins.

Cox, J., Campbell, A.V. and Fulford, B.K.W.M. (eds) (2007) *Medicine of the Person.* London: Jessica Kingsley Publishers.

Craig, C. and Killick, J. (2004) 'Reaching Out with the Arts: Meeting with the Person with Dementia.' In A. Innes, C. Archibald and C. Murphy (eds) *Dementia and Social Inclusion.* New York: Jessica Kingsley Publishers.

Cuijpers, P., Van Straten, A. and Warmerdam, L. (2007) 'Behavioral activation treatments of depression: A meta-analysis.' *Clinical Psychology Review 27*, 3, 318–326.

Dalby, P., Sperlinger, D.J. and Boddington, S. (forthcoming) 'The lived experience of spirituality, religious faith and dementia in older people living with mild to moderate dementia.' *Dementia: The International Journal of Research and Practice.*

Damasio, A. (2003) *Looking for Spinoza: Joy, Sorrow and the Feeling Brain.* Orlando, FL: Harcourt Inc.

Davis, R. (1992) *My Journey into Alzheimer's Disease.* London: Tyndale.

de Caussade, J.-P. (1996) *The Sacrament of the Present Moment.* New York: Harper Collins.

Deleuze, G. and Guattari, F. (1972) *Anti-Œdipus.* London and New York: Continuum.

Dening, T. and Milne, A. (2009) 'Depression and mental health in care homes for older people.' *Quality in Ageing 10*, 1, 40–46.

Department of Health (2008) *IAPT Implementation Plan: National Guidelines for Regional Delivery.* Available at http://www.dh.gov.uk/prod_consum_dh/groups/dh_digitalassets/@dh/@en/documents/digitalasset/dh_083168.pdf, accessed on 24 February 2011.

Deveson, A. (2003) *Resilience.* Sydney: Allen and Unwin.

Donne, J. (1987) 'Seventh Meditation.' In A. Raspa (ed.) *Devotions Upon Emergent Occasions.* New York: Oxford University Press. First published 1624.

Doubleday, E.K., King, P. and Papageorgiou, P. (2002) 'Relationship between fluid intelligence and ability to benefit from cognitive behavioural therapy in older adults: A preliminary investigation.' *British Journal of Clinical Psychology 41*, 423–428.

D'Souza, R. (2007) 'The importance of spirituality in medicine and its application in clinical practice.' *Medical Journal of Australia 186*, S57–59.

Ecclesiasticus (1970) 'Ecclesiasticus or the Wisdom of Jesus Son of Sirach.' In *The New English Bible.* Oxford and Cambridge: Oxford and Cambridge University Presses.

Ekers, D., Richards, D. and Gilbody, S. (2008) 'A meta-analysis of randomized trials of behavioural treatment of depression.' *Psychological Medicine 38*, 5, 611–623.

Ellor, J.W., Stetner, J. and Spath, H. (1987) 'Ministry with the confused elderly.' *Journal of Religion and Ageing 4*, 2, 21–33.

Engel, G.L. (1980) 'The clinical application of the biopsychosocial model.' *American Journal of Psychiatry 137*, 5, 535–544.

Erikson, E.H. (1977) *Toys and Reasons: Stages in the Ritualization of Experience.* New York: W.W. Norton.

Erikson, E.H. (1982) *The Life Cycle Completed: A Review.* London: W.W. Norton.

Erikson, J.M. (1995) *On Old Age. 1: A Conversation with Joan Erikson at 90.* San Luis Obispo, CA: Davidson Films. [Video]

Erikson, J.M. (1997) *The Life Cycle Completed: Extended Version with New Chapters on the Ninth Stage of Development.* New York and London: W.W. Norton & Company.

Everett, D. (1996) *Forget Me Not: The Spiritual Care of People with Alzheimer's.* Edmonton: Inkwell Press.

Feil, N. (1982) *Validation: The Feil Method.* Cleveland, OH: Edward Feil Productions.

Fleming, R. (2001) *Challenge Depression Programme.* Canberra: Commonwealth Department of Health and Ageing.

Folland, M. (2005) 'Caring for the spirit.' *Nursing Management 12*, 6, 20.

Frank, A. (undated) *Notes on Habermas: Lifeworld and System.* Available at http://people.ucalgary.ca/~frank/habermas.html, accessed on 24 February 2011.

Frankl, V. (1984) *Man's Search for Meaning.* New York:Washington Square Press.

Friedan, B. (1993) *The Fountain of Age.* New York: Simon and Schuster.

Froggatt, K. and Moffitt, L. (1997) 'Spiritual needs and religious practice in dementia care.' In M. Marshall (ed.) *State of the Art in Dementia Care.* London: Centre for Policy on Ageing.

Gibson, F. (1999) 'Can we risk person-centred communication?' *Journal of Dementia Care 7*, 5, 22–24.

Gilbert, P. (ed.) (2005) *Compassion: Conceptualisations, Research and Use in Psychotherapy.* London and New York: Routledge.

Gilbert, P. (2009) *The Compassionate Mind.* London: Constable.

Gillies, A. (2009) *Keeper.* London: Short Books.

Goldsmith, M. (1996) *Hearing the Voice of People with Dementia: Opportunities and Obstacles.* London: Jessica Kingsley Publishers.

Goldsmith, M. (1999) 'Dementia: a Challenge to Christian Theology and Pastoral Care.' In A. Jewell (ed.) *Spirituality and Ageing.* London: Jessica Kingsley Publishers.

Goldsmith, M. (2004) *In a Strange Land: People with Dementia and the Local Church.* Southwell: 4M Publications.

Goodall, M. (2009) 'The evaluation of spiritual care in a dementia care setting.' *Dementia 8,* 2, 167–183.

Goodall, M. (2010) 'Meeting the Needs of a Person with Dementia in a Care Home.' In J. Woodward (ed.) *Between Remembering and Forgetting.* London: Continuum Mobray.

Gooder, P. (2009) *The Risen Existence: The Spirit of Easter.* London: Canterbury Press.

Graham, S., Hampshire, A., Hindmarsh, E., Squires, B. and Wall, S. (2004). *My Health, My Future, My Choice: An Advance Care Directive for New South Wales.* Available at www.advancedorectives.org.au, accessed on 21 November 2010.

Green, P. (2006) 'CBT: The treatment of choice for older adults with mental health problems.' *Nursing Minds,* Winter/Spring, 4–5.

Green, P. (2007) 'Adapting CBT using a compassionate mind approach with older people who experience dementia and depression.' *PSIGE Newsletter 99,* 5–8.

Gubrium, J.F. (1986) 'The social preservation of mind: The Alzheimer's disease experience.' *Symbolic Interaction 9,* 1, 37–51.

Habermas, J. (1984, 1987) *The Theory of Communicative Action. Vols. 1 and 2.* Boston, MA: Beacon.

Hammond, G. (1999) *The Friendship Club.* Leeds: Faith in Elderly People.

Hammond, G. (2000) *The Memory Box.* Leeds: Faith in Elderly People.

Hammond, G. (2009) *Training Manual for Care Homes.* Leeds: Faith in Elderly People.

Hammond, G. and Moffitt, L. (2000) *Spiritual Care: Guidelines for Care Plans.* Leeds: Faith in Elderly People and Christian Council on Ageing.

Hammond, G. and Owen, S. (2006) *Safe to Belong.* Didcot: Baptist Union of Great Britain.

Hammond, G. and Treetops, J. (2004) *Wells of Life.* Leeds: Faith in Elderly People.

Hanh, T.N. (2009) *Calendar California.* Ann Arbor, MI: Brush Dance.

Harrington, A. (2010a) 'Ageing and Spirituality: Living and Being in Multifaith and Multicultural Communities.' In E. MacKinlay (ed.) *Ageing and Spirituality across Faiths and Cultures.* London: Jessica Kingsley Publishers.

Harrington, A. (2010b) 'Spiritual Well-being for Older People.' In E. MacKinlay (ed.) *Ageing and Spirituality across Faiths and Cultures.* London: Jessica Kingsley Publishers.

Harris, J. (1998) 'Spirituality in the Later Years of Life.' In A. Jewell (ed.) *Age Awareness Pack* (Booklet 1). Derby: Methodist Homes for the Aged and Christian Council on Ageing.

Harris, J. (2003) 'In praise of unprincipled ethics.' *Journal of Medical Ethics 29,* 5, 303–306.

Hauerwas, S. (1988) *Taking Time for Peace. Christian Existence Today.* Durham, NC: Labyrinth Press.

Hawley, G. and Jewell, A. (2009) *Crying in the Wilderness.* Derby: MHA.

Hay, D. (2006) *Something There: The Biology of the Human Spirit.* London: Darton Longman and Todd.

Hay, D. and Nye, R. (2006) *The Spirit of the Child.* London: Jessica Kingsley Publishers.

Heidegger, M. (1962) *Being and Time* (transl. J. Macquarrie and E. Robinson). Malden, MA, Oxford and Carlton, Australia: Blackwell.

Henderson, C.S. and Andrews, N. (1998) *Partial View: An Alzheimer's Journal.* Dallas, TX: Southern Methodist University Press.

Hepple, J. (2004) 'Psychotherapies with older people: An overview.' *Advances in Psychiatric Treatment,* 10, 371–377.

Hepworth, M. (2000) *Stories of Ageing.* Buckingham : Open University Press.

Higginson, G. (2006) 'Compassionate mind training for individuals who experience shame and self attacking related to their experience of early onset dementia syndrome.' Presentation given at The Rampant Lion Pub, Manchester, 16 June 2006.

Hill, P.C. and Pargament, K.I. (2003) 'Advances in the conceptualization and measurement of religion and spirituality: Implications for physical and mental health research.' *American Psychologist 58*, 1, 64–74.

Hilton, C. (2009) 'The East Riding of Yorkshire improving access to psychological therapies pathfinder project: Struggles in relation to the inclusion of older people.' *PSIGE Newsletter 106*, 26–30.

Holy Bible, New International Version (1973, 1978, 1984). Colorado Springs, CO: International Bible Society.

Hughes, J.C. (2001) 'Views of the person with dementia.' *Journal of Medical Ethics 27*, 2, 86–91.

Hughes, J.C. (ed.) (2006) *Palliative Care in Severe Dementia.* London: Quay Books.

Hughes, J.C. (2008) 'Being Minded in Dementia: Persons and Human Beings.' In M. Downs and B. Bowers (eds) *Excellence in Dementia Care.* Buckingham: Open University Press/McGraw Hill.

Hughes, J.C., Lloyd-Williams, M. and Sachs, G.A. (eds) (2010) *Supportive Care for the Person with Dementia.* Oxford: Oxford University Press.

Hughes, J.C., Louw, S.J. and Sabat, S.R. (eds) (2006) *Dementia: Mind, Meaning, and the Person.* Oxford: Oxford University Press.

Huizinga, J. (1955) *Homo Ludens: A Study of the Play Element in Culture.* Boston, MA: Beacon Press.

Hyde, B. (2008) *Children and Spirituality: Searching for Meaning and Connectedness.* London: Jessica Kingsley Publishers.

Ignatieff, M. (1992) 'A taste of ice-cream is all you know.' *The Observer*, 4 July.

Innes, A. (2009) *Dementia Studies: A Social Science Perspective.* London: Sage.

James, I.A. (2003) 'Working with older people: Implications for schema theory.' *Clinical Psychology and Psychotherapy 10*, 133–143.

James, I.A., Kendell, K. and Reichelt, F.K. (1999) 'Conceptualisation of depression in older people: The interaction of positive and negative beliefs.' *Behavioural and Cognitive Psychotherapy 27*, 3, 285–290.

Jewell, A. (ed.) (1999) *Spirituality and Ageing.* London: Jessica Kingsley Publishers.

Jewell, A. (ed.) (2004) *Ageing, Spirituality and Well-being.* London: Jessica Kingsley Publishers.

Jewell, A. (2004) 'Nourishing the Inner Being: A Spiritual Model.' In A. Jewell (ed.) *Ageing, Spirituality and Well-being.* London: Jessica Kingsley Publishers.

Jewell, A. (2009) 'Spirituality and ageing.' *The Newman: The Journal of the Newman Association 77*, 2–7.

Jewell, A. (2010) 'The importance of purpose in life in an older British Methodist sample: Pastoral implications.' *Journal of Religion, Spirituality and Aging 22*, 3, 138–162.

Jones, C. (1989) *The Search for Meaning.* Sydney: ABC Books.

Jung, C.G. and Read, H. (1960) *The Collected Works of C.G. Jung, Vol. I: The Structure and Dynamics of the Psyche.* London: Routledge and Kegan Paul.

Kabat-Zinn, J. (1994) *Mindfulness Meditation for Everyday Life.* London: Piatkus.

Kabat-Zinn, J. (2005) *Full Catastrophe Living: Using the Wisdom of Your Body and Mind to Face Stress, Pain and Illness.* New York: Bantam Dell.

Kemp, P. and Wells, P. 'Spirituality in healthcare: What can you do?' *British Journal of Healthcare Assistants 3*, 7, 333–337.

Kennison, P. (1990) 'Taking time for the trivial: Reflections on yet another book from Hauerwas.' *Asbury Theological Journal 45*, 1, 65–74.

Killick, J. (1997) 'Communication: A matter of the life and death of the mind.' *Journal of Dementia Care 5*, 5, 14–15.

Killick, J. (2004) *Dementia Poems.* London: Hawker Publications.

Killick, J. (2006) 'Helping the flame to stay bright: Celebrating the spiritual in dementia.' *Journal of Religion, Spirituality and Aging 18*, 2/3, 73–78.

Kimble, M. (2001) 'A Personal Journey of Aging: The Spiritual Dimension.' In S.H. McFadden and R.C. Atchley (eds) *Aging and the Meaning of Time.* New York: Springer Publishing Co.

Kimble, M.A. and Ellor, J.W. (2000) 'Logotherapy: An Overview.' In M. Kimble (ed.) *Viktor Frankl's Contribution to Spirituality and Aging.* Binghampton, NY: The Haworth Pastoral Press.

King, U. (2004) 'The Dance of Life: Spirituality, Ageing and Human Flourishing.' In A. Jewell (ed.) *Ageing, Spirituality and Well-being.* London: Jessica Kingsley Publishers.

Kitwood, T. (1990) 'Understanding senile dementia: A psychobiographical approach.' *Free Associations 19*, 60–76.

Kitwood, T. (1993) 'Towards a theory of dementia care: The interpersonal process.' *Ageing and Society 13*, 51–67.

Kitwood, T. (1995) 'Positive long-term changes in dementia: Some preliminary observations.' *Journal of Mental Health 1*, 2, 133–144.

Kitwood, T. (1997a) *Dementia Reconsidered: The Person Comes First.* Buckingham: Open University Press.

Kitwood, T. (1997b) 'Personhood, Dementia and Dementia Care.' In S. Hunter (ed.) *Dementia Challenges and New Directions.* London: Jessica Kingsley Publishers.

Kitwood, T. (1997c) 'The Concept of Personhood and its Relevance for a New Culture of Dementia Care.' In B.M.L. Miesen and G.M.M. Jones (eds) *Caregiving in Dementia: Research and Applications* (Volume 2). London: Routledge.

Kitwood, T. and Bredin, K. (1992a) 'Towards a theory of dementia care: Personhood and well-being.' *Ageing and Society 12*, 269–287.

Kitwood, T. and Bredin, K. (1992b) *Person to Person.* Loughton: Gale Centre Publications.

Knocker, S. (2010) 'Snapshots in Time: Time to Look out of the Window.' In J. Gilliard and M. Marshall (eds) *Time for Dementia: A Collection of Writings on the Meanings of Time and Dementia.* London: Hawker Publications.

Koenig, H.G. (1994) *Aging and God: Spiritual Pathways to Mental Health in Midlife and Later Years.* New York: Haworth Pastoral Press.

Koenig, H., McCullough, M. and Larson, D. (2001) *Handbook of Religion and Health.* Oxford: Oxford University Press.

Kontos, P.C. (2004) 'Ethnographic reflections on selfhood, embodiment and Alzheimer's disease.' *Ageing and Society 24*, 6, 829–849.

Lachlan, G. (2007) *On Meeting the Needs of Religious and Belief Communities within the Scottish NHS.* Interfaith Community Council. Edinburgh: Scottish Executive.

Lachlan. G. (2010) *Spiritual Needs, Health and Wellbeing.* Presentation to the University of the West of Scotland, Paisley, Summer 2010.

Laidlaw, K. (2001) 'An empirical review of cognitive therapy for late life depression: Does research evidence suggest adaptations are necessary for cognitive therapy with older adults?' *Clinical Psychology and Psychotherapy 8*, 1–14.

Laidlaw, K., Thompson, L.W., Dick-Siskin, L. and Gallagher-Thompson, D. (2003) *Cognitive Behaviour Therapy with Older People.* Chichester: Wiley.

Laidlaw, K., Thompson, L.W. and Gallagher-Thompson, D. (2004) 'Comprehensive conceptualisation of cognitive behaviour therapy for late life depression.' *Behavioural and Cognitive Psychotherapy 32*, 4, 389–399.

Langdon, S.A., Eagle, A. and Warner, J. (2007) 'Making sense of dementia in the social world: A qualitative study.' *Social Science and Medicine 64*, 989–1000.

Langer, E. (music) and Maxwell, G. (words) (2010) *The Lion's Face.* London: Oberon Modern Plays.

Larson, D.B., Sawyers, J.P. and McCullough, M. (1997) *Scientific Research on Spirituality and Health: A Consensus Report.* Rockville, MD: National Institute for Healthcare Research.

Lavretsky, H. (2003) 'Therapy of depression in dementia.' *Expert Review of Neurotherapeutics 3*, 5, 631–639.

Levinas, E. (1961) *Totality and Infinity.* Pittsburgh, PA: Duquesne University Press.

Lipinska, D. (2009) *Person-Centred Counselling for People with Dementia.* London: Jessica Kingsley Publishers.

Lloyd, M. (2003) 'Challenging depression: Taking a spiritually enhanced approach.' *Geriaction 21*, 4, 26–29.

Lloyd, M. (2004) 'Understanding spirituality: Tuning in to the inner being.' *Journal of Dementia Care 12*, 4, 25–27.

Lloyd, M. (2006) 'Resilience promotion and its role in clinical medicine.' *Australian Family Physician 35,* 12, 63–64.

Luntley, M. (2003) *Wittgenstein: Meaning and Judgement.* Malden, MA, Oxford and Carlton: Blackwell Publishing.

MacIntyre, A. (1985) *After Virtue: A Study in Moral Theory.* London: Duckworth.

MacKinlay, E. (2010) 'Ageing and Spirituality: Living and Being in Multifaith and Multicultural Communities.' In E. MacKinlay (ed.) *Ageing and Spirituality across Faiths and Cultures.* London: Jessica Kingsley Publishers.

MacKinlay, E., Trevitt, C. and Coady, M. (2002–2005) *Finding Meaning in the Experience of Dementia: The Place of Spiritual Reminiscence.* Australian Research Council Linkage Project, # LP0214980.

MacKinlay, E., Trevitt, C. and Hobart, S. (2002) *The Search for Meaning: Quality of Life for the Person with Dementia.* Unpublished project report, February 2002. University of Canberra Collaborative Grant, 2001.

Macquarrie, J. (1972) *Paths in Spirituality.* London: SCM Press.

Mahoney, A., Pargament, K.I., Murray-Swank, A. and Murray-Swank, N. (2003) 'Religion and the sanctification of family relationships.' *Review of Religious Research 1,* 149–162.

Martell, C.R., Addis, M.E. and Jacobson, N.S. (2001) *Depression in Context: Strategies for Guided Action.* New York: Norton.

Maslow, A.H. (1943) 'A theory of human motivation.' *Psychological Review 50,* 4, 370–396.

Matthews, E. (2002) *The Philosophy of Merleau-Ponty.* Chesham: Acumen.

McCabe, H. (1987) *God Matters.* London and New York: Mowbray.

McCloskey, L.J. (1990) 'The silent heart sings.' *Generations: Counselling and Therapy,* Winter 1990.

McFadden, S.H. (2004) 'The Paradoxes of Humor and the Burdens of Despair.' In E. MacKinlay (ed.) *Spirituality of Later Life: On Humor and Despair.* New York: Haworth Press.

McFadden, S.H. and Basting, A.D. (2010) 'Healthy aging persons and their brains: Promoting resilience through creative engagement.' *Clinics in Geriatric Medicine 26,* 1, 149–162.

McFadden, S.H., Frank, V. and Dysert, A. (2008) 'Creativity in the "now" of glimpses of the lifeworld in advanced dementia through storytelling and painting.' *Journal of Aging, Humanities, and the Arts 2,* 2, 135–149.

McFadyen, A. (1990) *The Call to Personhood.* Cambridge: Cambridge University Press.

McGinn, L.K. and Sanderson, W.C. (2001) 'What allows cognitive behavioural therapy to be brief: Overview, efficacy and crucial factors facilitating brief treatment.' *Clinical Psychology: Science and Practice 8,* 1, 23–27.

McGowin, D.F. (1993) *Living in the Labyrinth: A Personal Journey through the Maze of Alzheimer's.* Cambridge: Mainsail Press.

McLean, A. (2007) 'Dementia care as a moral enterprise: A call for a return to the sanctity of lived time.' *Alzheimer's Care Today 8,* 4, 360–372.

McRuer, R. (2006) *Crip Theory: Cultural Signs of Queerness and Disability.* New York: New York University Press.

Menne, H.L., Kinney, J.M. and Morhardt, D.J. (2002) 'Trying to continue to do as much as they can do: Theoretical insights regarding continuity and meaning making in the face of dementia.' *Dementia 1,* 367–382.

Mental Welfare Commission for Scotland (2009) *Remember I'm Still Me.* Edinburgh and Dundee: The Mental Welfare Commission for Scotland and Care Commission.

Merton, T. (1961) *New Seeds of Contemplation.* New York: New Directions Books.

MHA Care Group (2002) 'Nourishing the Inner Being' [videotape]. Derby: MHA.

MHA/CCOA (2006) *Worship with People with Dementia.* Derby: Methodist Homes for the Aged and Christian Council on Ageing.

MHA/CCOA (2008) *Visiting People with Dementia.* Derby: Methodist Homes for the Aged and Christian Council on Ageing.

Moberg, D. (1979) *Spiritual Well-Being: Sociological Perspective.* Lanham, MD: University Press of America.

Moltmann, J. (1974) *The Crucified God.* London: SCM Press.

Mowat, H. (2004) 'Successful Ageing and the Spiritual Journey.' In A. Jewell (ed.) *Ageing, Spirituality and Well-being.* London: Jessica Kingsley Publishers.

Mowat, H. (2007) *The Potential for Efficacy of Healthcare Chaplaincy – Spiritual Care Provision in the NHS (UK): A Scoping Review.* Sheffield: South Yorkshire NHS Strategic Health Board.

Mullan, M. and Killick, J. (2001) *Responding to Music* [book and videotape]. Stirling: Dementia Services Development Centre.

Muncey, T. (2005) 'Doing autoethnography.' *International Journal of Qualitative Method 4,* 1, 1–20.

Myers, F., McCollam, A. and Woodhouse, A. (2005) *Equal Minds: National Programme for Improving Mental Health and Wellbeing.* Edinburgh: Scottish Executive.

NHS Health Scotland (2004) *Mental Health and Wellbeing in Later Life: Older People's Perceptions.* Edinburgh: NHS Health Scotland.

NHS Health Scotland (2005) *Shifting the Balance of Care.* Edinburgh: NHS Health Scotland. Available at www.shiftingthebalance.scot.nhs.uk, accessed on 7 August 2010.

Nicholson, T. (1994) *Black Daisies for a Bride.* London: Faber and Faber.

O'Connor, D., Phinney, A., Smith, A., Small, J. *et al.* (2007) 'Personhood in dementia care.' *Dementia 6,* 121–142.

O'Connor, D. and Purves, B. (eds) (2009) *Decision-Making, Personhood and Dementia.* London: Jessica Kingsley Publishers.

Palazzini, L. (1994) 'Personalism and bioethics.' *Ethics and Medicine: An International Christian Perspective on Bioethics 10,* 1, 7–11.

Palo-Bengtsson, L. and Ekman, S.-L. (2002) 'Emotional response to social dancing and walks in persons with dementia.' *American Journal of Alzheimer's Disease and Other Dementias 17,* 3, 149–153.

Pargament, K.I. (2002) 'The bitter and the sweet: An evaluation of the costs and benefits of religiousness.' *Psychological Inquiry 13,* 3, 168–181.

Pargament, K.I. and Mahoney, A. (2005) 'Sacred matters: Sanctification as a vital topic for the psychology of religion.' *International Journal for the Psychology of Religion 13,* 3, 179–198.

Parry, B. (2009) 'Conveying compassion through attention to the essential ordinary.' *Nursing Older People 21,* 6, 14–21.

Pattison, S. (1988) *A Critique of Pastoral Care.* London: SCM Press.

Peterson, B. (2004) *Voices of Alzheimer's: Courage, Humor, Hope and Love in the Face of Dementia.* Cambridge, MA: De Capo Books.

Petzch, H. (1984) '"Does he know how frightening he is in his strangeness?" A study in attitudes to dementing people.' Edinburgh: University of Edinburgh Department of Practical Theology occasional paper.

Pinquart, M., Duberstein, P.R. and Lyness, J.M. (2007) 'Effects of psychotherapy and other behavioural interventions on clinically depressed older adults: A meta-analysis.' *Aging and Mental Health 11,* 6, 645–647.

Plummer, K. (1995) *Telling Sexual Stories: Power, Change and Social Worlds.* London: Routledge.

Pointon, B. (2007) 'The Search for Spirituality in Dementia: A Family Carer's Perspective.' In M.E. Coyte, P. Gilbert and V. Nicholls (eds) *Spirituality, Values and Mental Health: Jewels for the Journey.* London: Jessica Kingsley Publishers.

Post, S.G. (1995) *The Moral Challenge of Alzheimer Disease.* London: Johns Hopkins University Press.

Pruyser, P.W. (1968) *A Dynamic Psychology of Religion.* New York: Harper and Row.

Ramsey, A.M. (1969) *God, Christ and the World.* London: SCM Press.

Reinders, H. (2007) 'On Disability, Genetics and Choice.' In J. Swinton and B. Brock (eds) *Theology, Disability and the New Genetics: Why Science Needs the Church.* London: T. & T. Clark/Continuum.

Rhodes, B. (2005) 'Send in the clowns.' *Nursing Management 12,* 6, 13.

Ritzer, G. (2004) *The McDonaldization of Society.* Thousand Oaks, CA: Pine Forge Press.

Robbins, B.D. (2000) *Emmanuel Levinas.* Available at http://mythosandlogos.com/Levinas.html, accessed on 8 February 2011.

Robertson-Gillam, K. (2008) 'Hearing the Voice of the Elderly: The Potential for Choir Work to Reduce Depression and Meet Spiritual Needs: A Pilot Study.' In E. Mackinlay (ed.) *Ageing, Disability and Spirituality*. London: Jessica Kingsley Publishers.

Robinson, J.A.T. (1979) *Truth is Two-Eyed*. London: SCM Press.

Sacks, O. (1985) *The Man Who Mistook His Wife for a Hat and Other Clinical Tales*. London: Picador.

Sacks, O. (1998) 'Music and the Brain.' In C.M. Tomaino (ed.) *Clinical Applications of Music and Neurologic Rehabilitation*. St. Louis, MO: MMB Music Inc.

Sacks, O. (2007) *Musicophilia*. London: Picador.

Sapp, S. (2010) 'Spiritual Care of People with Dementia and their Carers.' In J.C. Hughes, M. Lloyd-Williams and G.A. Sachs (eds) *Supportive Care for the Person with Dementia*. Oxford: Oxford University Press.

Scholey, K.A. and Woods, B.T. (2003) 'A series of brief cognitive therapy interventions with people experiencing both dementia and depression: A description of techniques and common themes.' *Clinical Psychology and Psychotherapy 10*, 175–185.

Schotsmans, P. (1999) 'Personalism in medical ethics.' *Ethical Perspectives 6*, 1, 10–20.

Scottish Executive (2002a) *With Health in Mind*. Edinburgh: Scottish Executive.

Scottish Executive (2002b) *Health Directive Letter 76: Spiritual Care in Scotland*. Edinburgh: Scottish Executive.

Scottish Government (2007) *All Our Futures*. Available at www.scotland.gov.uk/Publications/2007/03/08125028/0, accessed on 24 February 2011.

Seligman, M.E.P. (2005) 'Positive Presentation and Positive Therapy.' In C.R. Synder and S.J. Lopez (eds) *Handbook of Positive Psychology*. Oxford: Oxford University Press.

Shamy, E. (1997) *More than Body, Brain and Breath: A Guide to the Spiritual Dimension of Care for People with Alzheimer's Disease*. Orewa: ColCom Press.

Shamy, E. (2003) *A Guide to the Spiritual Dimension of Care for People with Alzheimer's Disease and Related Dementias: More than Body, Brain and Breath*. London: Jessica Kingsley Publishers.

Shapiro, S.L., Carlson, L.E., Astin, J.A. and Freedman, B. (2006) 'Mechanisms of mindfulness.' *Journal of Clinical Psychology 62*, 3, 373–386.

Shouse, D. (2007) *Love in the Land of Dementia*. Kansas City, KS: Creative Connections.

Shults, F.L. and Sandage, S.J. (2006) *Transforming Spirituality: Integrating Theology and Psychology*. Grand Rapids, MI: Baker Academic.

Silcock, R. (1999) '46 Nursing Home' (play broadcast on BBC Radio 4).

Sixsmith, A., Stilwell, J. and Copeland, J. (1993) 'Rementia: Challenging the limits of dementia care.' *International Journal of Geriatric Psychiatry 8*, 12, 993–1000.

Small, N., Froggatt, K. and Downs, M. (2007) *Living and Dying with Dementia: Dialogues about Palliative Care*. Oxford: Oxford University Press.

Smith, H. (1958) *The Religions of Man*. New York: Harper and Row.

Smith, H. and Smith, M.K. (2008) *The Art of Helping Others: Being Around, Being There*. London: Jessica Kingsley Publishers.

Smith, J.A. (1997). 'Interpretive Phenomenological Analysis and the Psychology of Health and Illness.' In L. Yardley (ed.) *Material Discourses of Health and Illness*. London: Routledge.

Smith, J.A., Jarman, M. and Osborn, M. (1999) 'Doing Interpretive Phenomenological Analysis.' In M. Murray and K. Chamberlain (eds) *Qualitative Health Psychology: Theories and Methods*. London: Sage.

Smith, P. (1992) *The Emotional Labour of Nursing*. London: Macmillan.

Snowden, D. (2001) *Ageing with Grace*. New York: Bantam Books.

Snyder, L. (2002) *Speaking Our Minds: Personal Reflections from Individuals with Alzheimer's*. New York: W.H. Freeman.

South Yorkshire Strategic Health Authority (2003) *Caring for the Spirit*. Sheffield: South Yorkshire Strategic Health Authority.

Staffordshire University (D. Anderson and 18 other contributors) (2008) *A Collective Responsibility to Act Now on Ageing and Mental Health*. Available at www.staffs.ac.uk/assets/Collective_responsibility_to_act_now_on%20_ageing%20_and_mental_health_consensus_statement_tcm44-32411.pdf, accessed on 24 February 2011.

Stanworth, R. (2004) *Recognising the Spiritual Needs of People who are Dying.* Oxford: Oxford University Press.

Steindl-Rast, D. and Lebell, S. (2001) *Music of Silence: A Sacred Journey through the Hours of the Day* (quoted in Kemp and Wells 2009, p.334). Berkeley, CA: The Ulysses Press.

Stokes, G. (2000) *Challenging Behaviour in Dementia.* Bicester: Winslow.

Sturmey, P. (2009) 'Behavioural activation is an evidence-based treatment for depression.' *Behaviour Modification 33*, 6, 818–829.

Swinton, J. (2000) *Resurrecting the Person.* Nashville, TN: Abingdon Press.

Swinton, J. and Mowat, H. (2006) *Practical Theology and Qualitative Research Methods.* London: SCM Press.

Tacey, D. (2003) *The Spirituality Revolution: The Emergence of Contemporary Spirituality.* Sydney: HarperCollins.

Taylor, C. (1989) *Sources of the Self.* Cambridge: Cambridge University Press.

Teri, L. and Gallagher-Thompson, D. (1991) 'Cognitive-behavioural interventions for treatment of depression in Alzheimer's patients.' *The Gerontologist 31*, 3, 413–416.

Teri, L., Logsdon, R.G., Uomoto, J. and McCurry, S.M. (1997) 'Behavioural treatment of depression in dementia patients: A controlled clinical trial.' *Journal of Gerontology: Psychological Sciences 52B*, 4, 159–166.

TMK Productions and Memory Bridge (2007) *When Your Heart Wants to Remember* [film]. Extracts available at www.memorybridge.org, accessed on 14 February 2011.

Tournier, P. (1957) *The Meaning of Persons.* London: SCM Press.

Tournier, P. (1978) 'Relationships: The third dimension of medicine.' *Christian Medical Commission, Contact Bulletin 4.* Geneva: World Council of Churches.

Treetops, J. (1999) 'The Memory Box.' In A. Jewell (ed.) *Spirituality and Ageing.* London: Jessica Kingsley Publishers.

Trevitt, C. and MacKinlay, E. (2004) 'Just because I can't remember: Religiousness in older people with dementia.' *Journal of Religious Gerontology 16*, 3/4, 109–122.

Trevitt, C. and MacKinlay, E. (2006) 'I am just an ordinary person: Spiritual reminiscence in older people with memory loss.' *Journal of Religion, Spirituality and Aging 18*, 2/3, 77–89.

Ulverscroft (1974, 1989). *Large Print Song Books.* Leicester: F.A. Thorpe Publishing Ltd.

Vanier, J. (1989) *Community and Growth.* New York: Paulist Press.

Verkaik, R., Nuyen, J., Schellevis, F. and Francke, A. (2007) 'The relationship between severity of Alzheimer's disease and prevalence of co-morbid depressive symptoms and depression.' *International Journal of Geriatric Psychiatry 22*, 11, 1063–1080.

Vogler, S. (2003) *Dementia: The Loss…The Love…The Laughter.* Bloomington, IN: 1st Books.

Wainwright, D. (2001) *Being Rather than Doing.* Derby: Christian Council on Ageing.

Whitman, L (ed.) (2010) *Telling Tales about Dementia.* London: Jessica Kingsley Publishers.

Wittgenstein, L. (1968) *Philosophical Investigations* (eds G.E.M. Anscombe and R. Rhees; transl. Anscombe). Oxford: Blackwell.

Wittgenstein, L. (1974) *Tractatus Logico-Philosophicus* (transl. D.F. Pears and B.F. McGuiness). London and New York: Routledge.

Woods, B., Keady, J. and Seddon, D. (2008) *Involving Families in Care Homes.* London: Jessica Kingsley Publishers.

World Health Organization (2010) *WHO Definition of Palliative Care.* Geneva: World Health Organization. Available at www.who.int/cancer/palliative/definition/en, accessed on 24 September 2010.

Wuthnow, R. (2003) *All in Sync: How Music and Art are Revitalizing American Religion.* Berkeley, CA: University of California Press.

Young, W.M. (2007) *The Shack.* London: Hodder and Stoughton.

Žižek, S. (2006) *How to Read Lacan.* London: Granta.

SUBJECT INDEX

AUTHOR INDEX